PERSONALITY DISORDERS

DATE DUE

FEB 04 2020	
	PRINTED IN U.S.A.

PERSONALITY DISORDERS
A Practical Guide

Carol W. Berman, M.D.
Clinical Instructor in Psychiatry
New York University Medical Center
New York, New York

Wolters Kluwer Health | Lippincott Williams & Wilkins

Philadelphia · Baltimore · New York · London
Buenos Aires · Hong Kong · Sydney · Tokyo

5/25/10
Lan
$42.95

Acquisitions Editor: Charles W. Mitchell
Managing Editor: Sirkka E. Howes
Marketing Manager: Kimberly Schonberger
Production Editor: Beth Martz
Design Coordinator: Stephen Druding
Compositor: Spearhead Global, Inc.

Copyright © 2009 Carol W. Berman

Printed in China

9 8 7 6 5 4 3 2 1

Library of Congress Cataloging-in-Publication Data

Berman, Carol W.
   Personality disorders : a practical guide / Carol W. Berman.
      p. ; cm.
   Includes bibliographical references and index.
   ISBN 978-0-7817-9401-5
1. Personality disorders. I. Title.
   [DNLM: 1. Personality Disorders. 2. Psychotherapy—methods. WM 190 B516p 2009]
   RC554.B47 2009
   616.85'81—dc22

                                                                         2009003394

Care has been taken to confirm the accuracy of the information present and to describe generally accepted practices. However, the authors, editors, and publisher are not responsible for errors or omissions or for any consequences from application of the information in this book and make no warranty, expressed or implied, with respect to the currency, completeness, or accuracy of the contents of the publication. Application of this information in a particular situation remains the professional responsibility of the practitioner; the clinical treatments described and recommended may not be considered absolute and universal recommendations.

The authors, editors, and publisher have exerted every effort to ensure that drug selection and dosage set forth in this text are in accordance with the current recommendations and practice at the time of publication. However, in view of ongoing research, changes in government regulations, and the constant flow of information relating to drug therapy and drug reactions, the reader is urged to check the package insert for each drug for any change in indications and dosage and for added warnings and precautions. This is particularly important when the recommended agent is a new or infrequently employed drug.

Some drugs and medical devices presented in this publication have Food and Drug Administration (FDA) clearance for limited use in restricted research settings. It is the responsibility of the health care provider to ascertain the FDA status of each drug or device planned for use in their clinical practice.

To purchase additional copies of this book, call our customer service department at **(800) 638-3030** or fax orders to **(301) 223-2320**. International customers should call **(301) 223-2300**.

Visit Lippincott Williams & Wilkins on the Internet: http://www.lww.com. Lippincott Williams & Wilkins customer service representatives are available from 8:30 am to 6:00 pm, EST.

To Marty, for his love and support
To Rosemarie, for her dedication and work

Contents

Preface ix

Section I. The Personality Disorder

1. General Considerations 3
2. Paranoid Personality Disorder 7
3. Schizoid Personality Disorder 13
4. Antisocial Personality Disorder 17
5. Borderline Personality Disorder 21
6. Histrionic Personality Disorder 25
7. Narcissistic Personality Disorder 31
8. Avoidant Personality Disorder 35
9. Dependent Personality Disorder 39
10. Obsessive-Compulsive Personality Disorder 43
11. Personality Disorder, Not Otherwise Specified ... 47
12. Schizotypal Personality Disorder 51
13. Passive-Aggressive Personality Disorder 55
14. Self-Defeating Personality Disorder 59

Section II. Axis I Intersecting Axis II

15. Personality Disorders and Major Depression 65
16. Personality Disorders and Bipolar Disorder 71
17. Personality Disorders and Panic Attacks 77
18. Personality Disorders and Schizophrenia 83
19. Personality Disorders and Obsessive-Compulsive Disorder 89
20. Personality Disorders and ADHD 95
21. Personality Disorders and Dementia 99
22. Personality Disorders and Eating Disorders 105

Section III. Treatment Issues

23. Cluster A Clues 113

24. Cluster B Clues 119

25. Cluster C Clues 125

26. Gender Benders 131

27. It's Just Culture 137

28. Personality Disorders and Substance Abuse 141

29. Personality Disorders, PTSD, and Somatoform
Disorders 147

30. Personality Disorders and a Medical Condition . . . 155

31. Dimensional Models 161

32. Do They Ever Change? 167

Appendix 173

Bibliography 185

Index 187

Preface

The only patient who ever stormed out of my office without even seeing me was a woman with borderline personality disorder. The social worker who referred her for a medication evaluation was the one who told me the patient's diagnosis, but just hearing about the woman's behavior from my secretary could have led me to that conclusion. I was five minutes late, but to this new patient my tardiness was unconscionable, a slap in the face. She also complained to her social worker therapist that my office was dirty and the staff rude. My colleague, who'd been to my office several times, knew that none of this was true, but she wasn't surprised that her patient made these complaints and never saw me. We chalked it up to the patient having borderline personality disorder. And even though I understood, I still felt guilty. Later I learned that the patient felt abandoned and abused and didn't really want medicine. The social worker explained that this woman often felt abused since that was how her parents treated her.

Nevertheless, the negative experience was not easy to forget. I brought it up with colleagues and had to hear many similar stories before I felt better. In fact when psychiatrists talk shop, they'll often be discussing patients with personality disorders, like borderline. We have so many effective medications and psychotherapies against schizophrenia, major depression, panic disorder, and so on. However, our arsenals against personality disorders are limited and often ineffective. How often have brilliant clinicians written about innovative treatments for the borderline or the narcissist, yet we're still left empty-handed and disturbed by their behaviors in our hospitals, clinics, and offices. That call at 3 AM was probably from a borderline patient. Or how about a bill for several thousand dollars that the patient never paid? Again borderline personality disorder. You felt as if you were the worst doctor who ever existed? Borderline patient. The list goes on and on and doctors have many war stories to share.

Personality disorders are notoriously difficult to treat. It's as if the patient suited himself into ancient iron armor. Sure he's protected in there, but it makes it almost impossible to reach him. The personality, or way of dealing with the world, is rigid and maladaptive. Our patient may be clunking around in medieval armor while the rest of us are wearing shorts and T-shirts. He suited up a long time ago—as a teen, because it was the best way to deal with the "slings and arrows of misfortune" at the time. However, now the armor is inappropriate, a burden for the patient and an ordeal for everyone else. We want to help him remove the armor, but we wind up just shouting through a little hole he may open in the headpiece.

Categorizing patients into the various types of personality disorders is useful. To understand that a patient ran out of your office because she felt abandoned and enraged is invaluable information if you ever get the chance to meet her. Even if you never do, you'll be able to deal with your own feelings of guilt and helplessness. On the other hand, just viewing a patient as a category is dangerous. Since personality disordered individuals are so difficult, it's tempting to just leave them stuck in their armored suits, slap on some labels, and be satisfied.

In this book I will explain every category of personality disorder through real case histories and vignettes. You'll get a taste of who the people are underneath the armor.

THE PERSONALITY DISORDER

1 General Considerations

Essential Concepts

- A personality disorder is an inflexible, lasting pattern of thinking, feeling, and behavior.
- The pattern is different from what is expected from others in the patient's environment.
- Onset is in adolescence or in early adulthood.
- The disorder leads to impairment and is maladaptive.

> Those with a personality disorder do not feel anxiety about their maladaptive behavior.
> —Kaplan and Sadock's *Synopsis of Psychiatry*

People with personality disorders are stuck in certain ways of thinking and feeling about the world that cause them to act against themselves and others. Since they do not consider their behaviors problematic, they are mostly unmotivated to change. Many psychotherapists, who understand personality disorders, have little expectations of these patients. Psychiatrists are much more optimistic about treating depression, psychosis, and other Axis I disorders. To further discourage treatment, there is evidence that genetic factors are at play in all the personality disorders. Family histories reveal that schizotypal, borderline personality disorders as well as other personality disorders are inherited through the generations. Of course, environment contributes to reinforcing paranoia and other defenses.

CLASSIFICATIONS

At present, we identify 10 specific personality disorders, one general category and two criteria sets that need further study.

1. *Paranoid Personality Disorder* is a pattern of distrust and suspicion in which other people are seen as malevolent.
2. *Schizoid Personality Disorder* is a pattern of detachment from others with a restricted emotional range.
3. *Schizotypal Personality Disorder* is a pattern of terrible discomfort in relationships with distortions of thinking and perceptions.
4. *Antisocial Personality Disorder* is a pattern of violations of other people's rights.
5. *Borderline Personality Disorder* is a pattern of instability of self and dealing with others.
6. *Histrionic Personality Disorder* is a pattern of excessive emotion and need for attention.
7. *Narcissistic Personality Disorder* is a pattern of grandiosity, lack of empathy, and need for admiration.
8. *Avoidant Personality Disorder* is a pattern of being socially inhibited due to fear of negative evaluation.
9. *Dependent Personality Disorder* is a pattern of needing to be cared for to the point in which the patient clings to others.
10. *Obsessive-Compulsive Personality Disorder* is a pattern of being over-involved with control and perfection.
11. *Passive-Aggressive Personality Disorder* is a pattern that needs further research, but it consists of negative attitudes and passive resistance.
12. *Self-Defeating Personality Disorder* is a pattern that needs further research, but consists of a patient acting against him-or-herself.
13. *Personality Disorder, Not Otherwise Specified* is a grab bag category for personality disorders that do not exactly fit into the other categories.

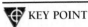 **KEY POINT**

All personality disorders are diagnosed under Axis II. It is important to remember to consider what clinical disorders (or Axis I) personality-disordered patients have.

To make diagnosis simpler the personality disorders have been clustered into three groups:

- *Cluster A* (the strange ones)
  Paranoid
  Schizoid
  Schizotypal
- *Cluster B* (the dramatic ones)
  Antisocial
  Borderline
  Histrionic
  Narcissistic
- *Cluster C* (the anxious ones)
  Avoidant
  Dependant
  Obsessive-Compulsive

 KEY POINT

Personality *traits* are not personality disorders. Traits are normal, adaptive patterns of relating to the environment. Only when they become entrenched and cause distress do they become disorders.

CLINICAL VIGNETTE

A 37-year-old attorney came to visit me for the first time. She chose to sit in a chair that faced away from the window, even though my floor-length curtains were fully drawn.

Before I could even begin her session she insisted that I follow strict rules for addressing her. I was not to call her by her first name, but instead Ms. X. She wanted a copy of my notes as soon as possible. Also, she wanted me to sign two of her own forms, indicating that I would not share any information about her with other therapists or insurance companies.

I complied with her wishes, but immediately began to consider a personality disorder as part of her diagnosis.

Ms. X needed to control the interview as much as possible because she was inflexible. This maladaptive pattern had started in early adulthood. Her pervasive suspicions about everyone caused people to stay away from her and she believed their reaction meant that they were malevolent. Her assumption, before she knew me, was that I would betray or harm her. My diagnosis was Axis II Paranoid Personality Disorder as well as major depression on Axis I.

The lasting patterns of personality disorders extend across a broad range of situations and lead to distress and impairment of interactions. When making the diagnosis of a personality disorder, you have to be careful to rule out substance abuse and medical conditions that might make you suspect that you are dealing with a personality-disordered patient.

2

Paranoid Personality Disorder

Essential Concepts

- Your Paranoid Personality Disorder (PPD) patients think everyone is out to harm them. Trust is limited.
- PPD patients are suspicious of their sexual partners and doubt the loyalty of everyone.
- PPD patients are unforgiving and read hidden meaning into simple situations.
- There is no or little reason for them to doubt, but they do.

Just because you're paranoid it doesn't mean someone's not out to get you.

—Unknown

Dealing with patients with Paranoid Personality Disorder (PPD) can be discouraging. No matter how hard you try to gain their trust, you probably will not succeed. They won't confide in you. Instead, the patient will suspect that you wish to deceive him or her. The most benign remarks can be misinterpreted as malicious. How hard it is to do psychotherapy or even dispense medications for them. Their hostility and anger get projected on to other people.

Many times we psychiatrists answer one question with another. The patient asks, "Where do you live?" We reply, "How is where I live relevant to your therapy?" Psychoanalysts, in particular, have been taught that every question reveals something about a patient and no question should be answered simply. However, when dealing with a PPD patient, to answer one question with another only leads the patient to more suspicion. Therefore, if your PPD patient asks the above question, reply with "I live in the neighborhood." To answer him directly may gain you some alliance. Of course, if he wants your exact address, you can tell him that would be inappropriate. Remember that patients unconsciously attempt to get you to feel the way they do. If you are feeling paranoid while treating your patient, you should start thinking about the diagnosis of PPD, and also rule out schizophrenia and other psychotic disorders.

 TIP

Always try to be as straightforward as possible with a PPD patient. If the patient comments on something he sees that is true, do not try to deny it.

CLINICAL VIGNETTE

Cindy, a 49-year-old, felt extreme pain in her abdomen one night. Before she called 911, she was determined to try every remedy, i.e., antacids, a hot water bottle, deep breathing. Finally, she gave up when nothing helped and allowed the ambulance to take her to the E.R. From there, she was rushed into the O.R. for an emergency appendectomy. The day after the successful operation, she asked her surgeon: "Are you sure I really needed that operation?" "I saved your life!" the surgeon responded, shocked at her question.

Cindy had another day to contemplate everything before they discharged her. During that time she questioned nurses and other staff suspecting that they had forced her into a needless procedure to get her insurance money. She was angry with everyone and threatened to sue the hospital.

Cindy's distrust and suspiciousness clearly landed her in the category of Paranoid Personality Disorder. If she had not been in such extreme pain she would have ignored her appendicitis to the point where it may have cost her life. By early adulthood, Cindy was convinced that people were out to exploit and deceive her. As a consequence, she stayed away from most people, except for a brief period in her twenties when she engaged in sexual relationships, but she constantly believed that her partners were unfaithful. She bore a grudge against the hospital and consulted an attorney to sue. He discouraged the suit by pointing out that no harm had come to her.

KEY POINT

If the patient is hallucinating, then he or she probably has schizophrenia, not PPD. PPD individuals may have brief psychotic episodes, but they rarely continue to be delusional or hallucinate.

The Axis I diagnosis may be Bipolar I Disorder, manic state, and your patient is seeing multicolored faces and hearing them talk. You prescribe the latest antipsychotic and in a week the patients stops hallucinating. Unfortunately, she remains suspicious of you and everyone else. You find out that she always has doubted other people and read hidden meanings into simple situations. In this case, you should write: Axis I: Bipolar I Disorder, manic state, Axis II: Paranoid Personality Disorder.

You cannot make your diagnosis of PPD or any other personality disorder as quickly as you can determine depression or psychosis. As you treat your patients over time and determine what patterns they are stuck in, you will be able to recognize the personality disorders.

DSMIV-TR wants a patient to have four or more of the following attributes to make the PPD diagnosis:

1. Suspects, without sufficient basis, that others are exploiting, harming, or deceiving him or her
2. Is preoccupied with unjustified doubts about the loyalty or trustworthiness of friends or associates
3. Is reluctant to confide in others because of unwarranted fear that the information will be used maliciously against him or her
4. Reads hidden demeaning or threatening meanings into benign remarks of events
5. Persistently bears grudges, i.e., is unforgiving of insults, injuries, or slights
6. Perceives attacks on his or her character or reputation that are not apparent to others and is quick to react angrily or to counterattack
7. Has recurrent suspicion, without justification, regarding fidelity of spouse or sexual partner.

 KEY POINT

PPD patients have extreme difficulty in engaging in personal and intimate relationships.

Many times when PPD patients present for treatment they are also suffering from an Axis I diagnosis such as major depression. The Axis I diagnosis may be so flagrant that the personality disorder is not immediately apparent. You treat the depression with an antidepressant and weekly psychotherapy. Then when your patient is finally sleeping and eating well and has a good mood, you notice that he or she is still suspicious and doubting. He still cannot or will not find a girlfriend or boyfriend or significant other. That is when you start suspecting a personality disorder on Axis II.

If he or she miraculously does try to date another person, be prepared for problems. You will hear complaints of how untrustworthy and exploitative everyone is. Your PPD patient is bound to be disillusioned and doubtful about his or her new friend. The most probable conclusion will be a break up and your patient isolating himself or herself again.

The workplace will prove difficult for most PPD patients, unless they can just sit at their computers and not interact with others. If they have to attend meetings, then they may feel that their coworkers are using them as scapegoats or implying negative things about them. They are bound to find hidden meanings in casual references. PPD patients do not easily forgive people and they may devise elaborate revenge plans. Advise them *not* to act on their plans. Instead you can help them with reality testing, by reviewing the details of their workplace conflicts, and pointing out where their paranoid thinking interfered with their ability to relate to people.

PPD is thought to occur in 0.5% to 2.5% of the general population. Frequently, these patients avoid psychiatrists because they are so reluctant to confide in anyone. They may present for treatment if they have anxiety, depression, or psychosis. Many bigots and cranks have suffered from PPD.

3   Schizoid Personality Disorder

Essential Concepts
- Your Schizoid Personality Disorder (SPD) patient prefers to be alone.
- Sex with others and most pleasures do not mean that much to them.
- Neither praise nor criticism will get you too far.
- They have flat affects and are cold to people, but it is not due to psychosis.

> I prefer to be alone.
>
> —Greta Garbo

Loners and the socially isolated are classic examples of Schizoid Personality Disorder (SPD). They often make good computer people and prefer staying away from others. Many SPD patients actually report that they have reduced sensations and do not appreciate sex and other pleasures like most individuals. Important life events, like marriage or death of family members, may pass by SPD people without their expression of any emotions.

Occupational functioning can also be impaired, because the person with SPD does not bond with others or fit into the workplace well. SPD may first appear in childhood and adolescence with poor grades, isolation, and being picked on by other children. The lack of bonding with others does not lead to loneliness in the SPD. They are basically asocial, although they may respond to first-degree family members. The feelings of others are a mystery to them. Sometimes, they just blend in to the background and are not noticed.

Avoid trying to push SPD patients into socializing too quickly, especially at the beginning of treatment. They will resist your pressure intensely and not believe that you have their best interests in mind. After many years of treating them, they may humor you and try to date someone or attend a party. Then they will complain that they wasted their time or that they were completely ignored. Of course, you will point out that the way they behaved, no eye contact with others, or a social smile or engagement in conversation did not help them any. They will not understand your suggestions. No matter how often you reinforce their interactions with others, they cannot be coerced into staying with others.

 KEY POINT

The Schizoid Personality-Disordered person may experience very brief psychotic disorders in stressful times, but if psychosis continues consider schizophrenia or bipolar disorder.

CLINICAL VIGNETTE

As Janet was such a naturally pretty blonde with pink cheeks and limpid blue eyes, no one ever suspected that she was a loner. Her boyfriend lived in California and she in New York. Sometimes, they would actually meet in person. Most of the communication was via e-mail. Janet liked it that way. But then her boyfriend found another woman closer to home.

Janet felt depressed, something she was not familiar with since most of the time she hardly felt anything. She sought treatment from a psychiatrist who prescribed sertraline 100 mg. The medicine made her feel better in 4 weeks. The doctor insisted that she have weekly psychotherapy as well. Two previous relationships had faded out because Janet ignored phone calls and e-mails. During therapy, she admitted that she had done the same thing with this boyfriend.

However, she said she did not want to break up with him. The psychiatrist suggested many ways that Janet could reopen the lines of communication. She agreed, but never followed any of the suggestions and dropped out of treatment.

DISCUSSION

Her psychiatrist would probably give Janet a diagnosis of SPD. She met the criteria of the DSMIV-TR, because she had a pervasive pattern of detachment from social relationships and a restricted range of expression of emotions in interpersonal settings that began in early adulthood as well as (1) not desiring or enjoying close relationships; (2) she usually chose solitary activities; (3) she had little interest in sex with anyone; and (4) she showed emotional coldness.

 KEY POINT

SPD patients are not considered weird. They appear normal and distant.

If your patient is just distant and solitary, but not strange in any way, you are probably dealing with an SPD. If he is weird, i.e., believes that a family of witches has moved in next door and that is why his TV does not work, then your patient probably has Schizotypal Personality Disorder or a psychotic disorder.

SPD is a threatened category because many practitioners consider the social isolation and emotional distancing of SPD as defenses rather than a personality disorder. SPD in childhood could be a predictor of schizophrenia. In a dimensional approach (see Chapter 31), a schizoid personality will score high on aloofness, suspiciousness, and introspection.

Many times, SPD patients consider everything an invasion of their private boundaries. For example, if a patient's mother or anyone came into his room, he found it too intrusive. After leaving home for college, he never contacted his parents again. When his mother or father called he pretended he was someone else and hung up. Then he changed his number. This SPD patient had a fantasy of watching his parents from a distance and perhaps sending them a gift of money. He was unable to engage in social relationships in school. After college, he took a job in the financial field and remained isolated from others. This patient viewed himself as extremely ugly and unfit for society, even though he looked perfectly normal and believed people who told him so. His reality testing was intact, but he had low self-esteem. Neither praise nor criticism affected him that much.

Most SPD patients will never have close relationships or respond to others. Their detachment from people and constricted affects qualify them for the diagnosis of SPD. In addition, SPD may have an increased prevalence in relatives of people with schizophrenia. SPD is at the healthier end of a spectrum that has schizophrenia at one end and personality disorders on the other.

4 Antisocial Personality Disorder

Essential Points
- Your Antisocial Personality Disorder (APD) patient will do whatever he wants when he wants to.
- He will lie and exploit everyone.
- You will find him impulsive, irritable, and aggressive.
- Do not leave your wallet or things of value lying around if you do not want to lose them.

There's a sucker born every second.

—Unknown

Antisocial Personality Disorder (APD) patients have been said to have psychopathy or sociopathy. Their sickness consists of not wanting to and not being able to follow the laws of society. They repeatedly break social norms and the law. Many of these patients have had conduct disorders since they were children. When psychiatrists are asked to treat APD patients, it is a thankless task, because this personality disorder is particularly intractable. Despite all our advances in psychopharmacology and psychotherapy, those with APD are best dealt with outside a medical setting.

APD patients are not just narcissistic in their pursuits but they are also impulsive, aggressive, and deceitful. They have a reckless disregard for themselves and others when it comes to safety. Once they do cause other people harm, they are able to rationalize or ignore the problems. Their superegos have lacunae in them, as our psychoanalysts would say.

KEY POINT

The APD patient does not feel he needs to conform to the rules.

APD patients usually know what the rules are, unlike autistic, psychotic, retarded, or demented patients. They chose not to obey the rules, or laws, the standards that most people live by, because they feel they are smarter than others. They do not need to be squeezed into norms. They enjoy figuring out ways around things, but they are not just creative, because if people are harmed along the way it means nothing to them.

CLINICAL VIGNETTE

Danny, a tall, well-built, 29-year-old, knew that women found him attractive. He and his friends hung around the bowling alley looking for opportunities. He met Pam, a 32-year-old accountant, there. He invited her to a movie and dinner at an expensive new restaurant. The day of their date, Danny dressed very well and used his last $10 to buy Pam red roses. The movie was a private screening, but Danny insisted his name was on the list as he walked in. The theater manager could not find his name anywhere, but since Danny was so charming, he let them in. After a lobster and champagne dinner, Danny said he had forgotten his credit card at home. Pam had to pay.

After 5 months of dating, Danny moved in with Pam. He borrowed money from her, promising to pay it back as soon as he received a check owed to him from work. Pam secretly viewed his e-mail one evening when he was out and discovered that Danny was not even working! She confronted him when he returned home. After he calmed her down, they had a long talk. He continued to con her for a few more months before she discovered that he had a jail record and a six-year-old son whom he had never supported. Pam finally made Danny move out.

DISCUSSION

Danny meets the criteria of the DSMIV-TR for APD. His pervasive pattern of disregard for and violation of the rights of others occurred since the age of 15, as indicated by three (or more) of the following:

(1) Failure to conform to social norms with respect to lawful behaviors, as indicated by repeatedly performing acts that are grounds for arrest
(2) Deceitfulness, as indicated by repeated lying, use of aliases, or conning others for personal profit or pleasure
(3) Impulsivity or failure to plan ahead
(4) Irritability and aggressiveness, as indicated by repeated physical fights or assaults
(5) Reckless disregard for safety of self or others
(6) Consistent irresponsibility, as indicated by repeated failure to sustain consistent work behavior or honor financial obligations
(7) Lack of remorse, as indicated by being indifferent to or rationalizing having hurt, mistreated, or stolen from another.

APD is common among first-degree relatives, and it is likely that Danny's father had it too. Danny's father was irresponsible and abusive, and his parents divorced when Danny was 10. His father never helped to support Danny when he went to live with his mother. APD is more prevalent in men than in women, with a prevalence of 3% in men and 1% in women. Psychotherapy is often not successful; however, self-help groups have been found to be helpful, if patients will agree to attend them. Medications may be used to control the anger, anxiety, and depressive elements associated with APD.

Psychostimulants are recommended for patients who have combined attention-deficit/hyperactivity disorder. APD must be distinguished from the other personality disorders and schizophrenia.

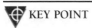 KEY POINT

Do not be fooled by the graciousness of your APD patients.

When interviewed, APD patients are amazingly composed and credible. Their charming and ingratiating manners often cover a tense, hostile interior ready to explode into sociopathy. If stressed during an interview, you may be able to glimpse some of the pathology underneath.

If you are fooled by an APD patient, realize that you are not the first one to succumb. The best way to handle it is to carry on with your patient's best interests in mind. This is not easy, because the patient does not have your best interests in his mind. He will not change, but you must maintain your integrity, even if you feel like getting even.

5   Borderline Personality Disorder

> **Essential Points**
> - Your Borderline Personality Disorder (BPD) patient will fight with everyone including you, due to inappropriate anger.
> - He or she will idealize or devalue people and have bad relationships in general.
> - Their unbalanced sense of self will include feelings of emptiness, fear of abandonment, and stress-induced dissociation.
> - Impulsivity will manifest as suicidal behavior, irritability, substance abuse, and over-spending.

> These patients must be considered to occupy a borderline area between neurosis and psychosis.
>
> —Otto Kernberg, M.D.

In the past, psychiatrists called Borderline Personality Disorder (BPD) patients the "as-if" personality or thought that they had "ambulatory" schizophrenia. They are some of the most difficult patients to treat because they can be so abusive to themselves and others, especially their therapists. A key to understanding them is to conceptualize their idealization and devaluation of others. They may think of you as an absolute "angel," who can do no wrong. In this idealized state you only have positive attributes, but in the next moment you can fall into a pit of devaluation and be conceived as a "devil" with only negative attributes. BPDs hardly ever see people as somewhere in the middle. We call this defense system "splitting." Because BPDs have such a distorted view of people, they often are angry, irritable, and anxious.

Their moods are highly reactive so they can swing from rage to paranoia to elation in minutes or hours, which is confusing to people dealing with them.

Impulsivity is another mark of a patient with BPD. They may suddenly slice their wrists, overdose on medications you have prescribed, or threaten to shoot themselves. They easily slip into substance abuse of one sort or another.

The best way to deal with patients with BPD is to set firm boundaries and try to maintain them. Time, place, and fees are to be enforced as strongly as you can. If you say you will be at the appointment at 10:30 a.m., do so. Try not to switch locations for your meeting, i.e., always meet in the same office if you can. Constantly monitor yourself for countertransference feelings, which you should do with all your patients but especially with these. If you are feeling angry, zero in on who the patient reminds you of, but be careful with interpretations. Patients with this personality disorder can barely withstand interpretations, especially if they are negative in any way.

 KEY POINT

Realize that your BPD patient may not improve. You are working hard to help your patients. You like to see some improvement. Do not expect it with BPD patients. If they do not decompensate further, you are doing a good job.

CLINICAL VIGNETTE

Paula, a 32-year-old medical intern, was constantly surprised by how quickly people changed. One minute she would adore a professor and the next minute despise him. She did not think there was anything wrong with her feelings. In the hospital where she interned, half the nursing staff thought Paula was the best intern and the other half detested her. Paula had started medical school later in life, having worked to save funds. At every job she had had horrendous fights with coworkers. Also in her marriage she had fought so much that she and her husband finally divorced. Paula felt lonely and abandoned by everyone, which drove her into indiscriminate, unprotected sex. She had a compulsive need for sex. Even though she was well aware that she should ask her partners to wear condoms, she did not. Instead she kept giving herself HIV tests. One night she felt horrible after trying to save a heart attack patient who died after 6 hours of intensive care. Both the nurses and the chief medical resident assured Paula that she had done an excellent job, but Paula could not stop berating herself. Alone in the on-call room she stormed into the bathroom and scraped a scalpel across her wrist. As soon as she saw her blood dripping she felt better. She cleaned and bandaged the superficial wound. Then she binge ate a giant bag of chocolate chip cookies.

DISCUSSION

Paula certainly fulfilled the DSMIV-TR criteria for BPD. She had an unstable self-image, seeing herself as extremely capable one minute and devalued the next minute. In a similar way, people with BPD either overidealize or devalue others, as Paula did with her professors and coworkers. Her interpersonal relationships were tense and unbalanced. When she was alone she felt empty, bored, and abandoned. Her inappropriate anger was taken out on herself when she sliced her wrist. Her impulsivity led to indiscriminate sex and binge eating.

Paula caused "splitting" of the staff at the hospital. Theorists have proposed that BPD patients view people as all good or bad, because they have failed to mentally integrate the "good mother" image with the "bad mother" image during infancy often because of abusive parenting. The "splitting" mechanism is used by an ego at regressed levels, where the mind can hold a good image far from a bad one, instead of incorporating the two.

 KEY POINT

BPD patients often feel entitled.

BPD patients will ask you and everyone else for special favors and expect to get them. If they do not, they may unleash anger at you or themselves. These patients must be treated with psychotherapy and often medications if they have depression or psychotic episodes. It is not advised to treat their anxiety with benzodiazepines because of BPD's tendencies toward addictions. Many clinicians use mood stabilizers.

Histrionic Personality Disorder

> I've always depended on the kindness of strangers.
> —Blanche DuBois in *A Streetcar Named Desire*,
> by Tennessee Williams

Histrionic Personality Disorder (HPD) is easy for the clinician to recognize, but like all personality disorders difficult to treat. HPD patients need to be the center of attention and their theatrical emotionality can be embarrassing. Often they are seductive in appearance and behavior. They impulsively seek excitement and novelty. The prevalence in the general population may only be 2% to 3%, but in our hospitals and clinics the percentage may be as high as 15%. Usually, women are diagnosed more than men, so that DSMV committees were reluctant to include the diagnosis for fear of sexual stereotyping. Sometimes, patients show fewer symptoms over the years. Perhaps they lose their energy or learn to control their behaviors.

The DSM IV-TR requires only five of the following criteria to make a diagnosis of HPD:

(1) The individual is uncomfortable in situations in which she is not the center of attention.
(2) Interaction with others is often characterized by inappropriate sexually seductive or provocative behavior.
(3) The individual displays rapidly shifting and shallow expression of emotions.
(4) The individual consistently uses physical appearance to draw attention to the self.
(5) The individual has a style of speech excessively impressionistic and lacking in detail.
(6) The individual shows self-dramatization, theatricality, and exaggerated expression of emotion.
(7) The individual is suggestible, easily influenced by others.
(8) The individual considers relationships more intimate than they actually are.

CLINICAL VIGNETTE

When I first met Suzie I was glad that I was not a man and did not have to steel myself against her provocative low-cut blouses and short skirts. She was a 5'10" slender redhead in her twenties, and I could see that many a male psychiatrist would have been distracted by her charms.

As I did with all my patients I maintained appropriate boundaries between us, by ending her sessions exactly on time and insisting that Suzie pay her fee each time. Suzie was not satisfied with such an arrangement. She would often try to extend sessions by telling me "the most exciting thing" two minutes before we had to end. Or she would often "forget" her check. I would reinforce that she had to adhere to our original arrangement and try to investigate why she felt the need to deviate. She enjoyed psychotherapy because she was clearly the center of attention. I did not respond to her oversexualized comments about me or her questions about my sex life, except to ask her what she thought about me to understand her transference. Her own sex life consisted of a series of one-night stands that she never found satisfying.

Suzie's chronic depression manifested itself in little sleep, decreased appetite, easy distractibility, irritability, and suicidal ideation. Our plan was to try to treat Suzie's depression with weekly psychoanalytical psychotherapy if we could. After several months, I saw that she was not progressing well and I suggested medication.

Suzie cried loudly, twisted around in her chair, and pleaded with me to reconsider.

Slowly and carefully I explained that the best option was pharmacotherapy. I was afraid that Suzie would decompensate further and perhaps attempt suicide if I withheld medication from her much longer.

"If you really think it will help me, I guess I'll try it," Suzie said dramatically. She crossed her legs in a slow way that revealed black lace panties under her short skirt. Any time I would interpret her seductive behavior she would completely deny its significance. Again I was happy to be a heterosexual woman, not swayed by her behavior. I wrote her a prescription for the antidepressant sertraline. "Start at 25 mg for three days. Then increase to 50 mg."

"Anything you say. We are such good friends, after all. How can I refuse you anything?"

Suzie believed what she said. I had asked her if she considered me a "friend" rather than her therapist or psychiatrist and she said yes. Interpretation of her feeling that I was a "friend" led nowhere. She also considered customers at her boutique, where she worked as a salesclerk, coworkers, her boss, one-night stands, and many other people her best friends. When she expressed this sentiment, many people would deny the friendship and then Suzie would cry.

 KEY POINT

Patients with personality disorders, which are diagnosed on Axis II, may also be depressed, anxious, or psychotic, diagnosed on Axis I.

Suzie displayed all eight of the criteria for HPD. She was uncomfortable at her boutique unless she was at the center of things. She tried to use her physical appearance to get attention from everyone and she was sexually seductive with me and others inappropriately. Her emotions shifted rapidly and her style of speech was exaggerated. When she was with me or her boyfriend she was suggestible. Finally, she considered me "such a good friend," when we only had a professional relationship. Suzie was not able to change her behavior according to circumstances. She was seductive even if people did not respond and it was inappropriate.

 KEY POINT

HPD patients are at an increased risk for suicide, but most of the time they just make gestures and threats to get more attention. Nevertheless, you should be careful in your assessment of risk.

CLINICAL VIGNETTE

At 11 p.m. one evening I received an emergency call from Suzie.

"I feel so nauseous. I'm sure I'll die," she declared.

"Take it easy, Suzie. Please tell me exactly what's wrong."

"There's this big bubble in my stomach. I feel as if I'll explode."

"Nausea is a common side effect with any of these medications. Just drink a ginger ale. I'm sure you'll feel better."

No matter how much I assured Suzie that she would be fine, she would not let me hang up. She sobbed and could not be reassured until I suggested that we meet in the emergency room where I could admit her for observation. She refused and finally let me get off the phone.

For the next few days, she called me daily to complain of nausea and a weird feeling in her head, even though she had stopped the antidepressant after one dose. When I finally saw her in the office, I asked for an explanation because she seemed about to launch into a different topic.

"The truth is I was with my boyfriend the first night I took the Zoloft. He kept telling me how bad antidepressants were for me. He said it would ruin our sex life." Suzie leaned forward showing her cleavage. "The more I talked to him, the worse I felt, until I was sure I would throw up, as I told you."

"How do you feel now?" I said quickly, before she could continue her monologue.

"I don't think I'll ever return to normal. I'm afraid I'm ruined for life."

I spent the next 20 minutes trying to explain to Suzie that one 25 mg tablet of the medication could not cause all the problems she described. By the end of the session she seemed to agree, but she never consented to take antidepressants again. After a few more weeks, she dropped out of treatment without receiving adequate care for her depression.

 KEY POINT

HPD patients may drop out of treatment precipitously if they are not constantly gratified.

What made Suzie have such an exaggerated and unusual response to such a tiny amount of medication?

Suzie had a nocebo reaction to the medication. Most doctors are familiar with a placebo, a sugar pill or any inert substance that has a positive effect on the patient. Not many are familiar with a nocebo, an inert substance that has a negative effect as a result of the patient's conscious or unconscious expectation of deterioration. Individuals with HPD are more likely to have either a placebo or nocebo effect to any small amount of medication because they are so suggestible. Negative transference, hopelessness, and helplessness all contribute to a nocebo effect. Suzie could just as easily have experienced a placebo effect, which would have enabled her to stay in treatment and benefit. Factors that would have favored a placebo effect would be positive transference, hopelessness, and a feeling that Suzie could be helped. Unfortunately, placebo and nocebo effects cannot be predicted or planned especially in HPD, in which the patient's emotions and transferences are rapidly shifting.

7 ▼ Narcissistic Personality Disorder

Essential Concepts

- Your Narcissistic Personality Disorder (NPD) patients will believe they are "special" and need your admiration.
- They will be grandiose and preoccupied with success fantasies.
- In their entitled way they are exploitative and lacking in empathy.
- Arrogance and envy are both abundant in NPD.

Narcissus kept staring into the pond, admiring himself, until he fell in and drowned.

—Greek myth

GREEK MYTHOLOGY

Narcissistic Personality Disorder (NPD) patients are entranced with themselves and expect others to feel the same. When most people do not, NPD patients become angry and arrogant in response to the world's indifference. They retreat into fantasies of perfect beauty, ideal love, and success. If someone is ill or has other needs, the NPD will ignore them and lack empathy about the person's problem. NPD is a chronic condition, which is notoriously difficult to treat. The disorder causes NPD patients to suffer more narcissistic injuries than others throughout their lives. For example, middle age and the entire aging process will be taken as injuries by NPD patients as they lose their looks, their jobs, and their family members. In many cases, they become envious of others.

⊕ KEY POINT

Do not try to convince an NPD patient that they are ordinary.

It may be hard to sympathize with an NPD patient who is so unsympathetic to everyone else. However, you must do your best to try to imagine yourself so blinded by your own image that no one else can exist. You will hear stories of your NPD patient sitting on the bus blabbing on the cell phone, oblivious to all, while a pregnant woman and an elderly, crippled man stand nearby. Never would your patient consider giving his seat to them. Do not lecture them about their lack of empathy; they will not get it. Also they will not continue treatment. It would be better to gently remind them to focus outward as an exercise to improve themselves. They are constantly seeking self-improvement.

Sometimes, clinicians find it difficult to distinguish between the narcissistic personality and the borderline personality. Both of these patients share entitled rage, but the NPD is enraged if someone threatens their superiority, while the BPD is enraged when their needs are not met and if they feel they are suffering.

CLINICAL VIGNETTE

Gloria, a single, attractive, 32-year-old woman, prided herself on taking excellent care of her body—especially her teeth, which were movie star white and perfectly straight. As a child, she had had many cavities, orthodontic work, and several teeth removed. Ever since adolescence, she focused obsessively on dental hygiene. To enhance her appearance further, Gloria dressed in the latest fashions and dyed her hair blonde. After experiencing minor pain in a front tooth, she visited her dentist, who informed her that it was so decayed it would need to be extracted. Gloria could not believe it! The tooth was pulled and Gloria had one complication after another, including bleeding gums, mouth sores, and pain. The emotional discomfort was even worse than the physical problems. Gloria could not stop thinking about the lost tooth; her tongue constantly touched the gap. She cried each morning when she scrutinized herself in the mirror. At night, she felt so depressed that she could not perform her usual activities. Her appetite decreased and she had difficulty sleeping. When Gloria's dentist suggested an implant, she hesitated to go through with it and instead went from one specialist to another trying to decide what to do. One day, while rushing around, she fell and lacerated her brow, which then required five stitches. Gloria could not tolerate looking at herself; a missing front tooth and a scarred face. It was too much. She refused to leave her house for several days. A cousin forced her to consult a psychiatrist who diagnosed major depression with obsessive features.

DISCUSSION

Gloria was placed on antidepressants, which cleared up her obsessions and depression. Her NPD could not be ameliorated so easily. She agreed to therapy with the psychiatrist. He explored her longest relationship, as well as her many short-term ones, and pointed out two important aspects of Gloria's social interactions. First, she was afraid of intimacy and never let friends get too close. When people asked about her parents or childhood, she would change the subject, afraid to reveal that her parents had been physically and emotionally abusive. She blocked her traumas. Second, she was arrogant, haughty, and angry when faced with other points of view. During a six-month relationship with a boyfriend, she fought constantly, attempting to achieve her goals at his expense. Gloria was encouraged to be more intimate with friends and try to entertain other viewpoints. Both goals were difficult for her.

KEY POINT

NPD patients will present for treatment for anxiety and depression.

Once the anxiety and depression have been treated with psychopharmacology and/or cognitive behavioral therapy, NPD will emerge. At that point you must work hard to have your patient continue in treatment. Do not expect them to relinquish their grandiose fantasies or decrease their special needs. Your empathy will amaze and delight them. That may be enough to maintain a therapeutic alliance.

8

Avoidant Personality Disorder

Essential Concepts
- Your Avoidant Personality Disorder (APD) patient fears interacting with others.
- APD patients believe that people will criticize and reject them.
- They feel inferior and inadequate.
- They avoid jobs, people, and new situations.

Why would he want to talk to me?
—Laura Wingfield in *The Glass Menagerie*,
by Tennesse Williams

Patients with Avoidant Personality Disorder (APD) are sure that other people will not like them, because they have such a bad opinion of themselves. Their schoolwork or jobs suffer because they constantly worry that people may criticize or reject them. They are hypervigilant about their environments, checking everyone's reactions to them. APD patients expect to be rejected, except when other people are extremely supportive and nurturing. The best way to treat these patients is to give them as much positive reinforcement as possible. APD patients will only trust you after many sessions in which you express positive regard for them. Unfortunately, they may avoid sessions in the beginning of treatment because they expect to be rejected.

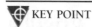 **KEY POINT**

APD patients may become intimate with people if they feel they are accepted unconditionally.

APD patients avoid people because they are so hypersensitive to rejection. Unlike schizotypal and schizoid patients they have more capacity for relationships, but they are so fearful that others will ridicule them. People see them as shy and self-effacing. In the workplace, they seldom become supervisors and often work in positions far below their abilities. When clinicians first interview these patients, they are anxious and have difficulty talking about themselves. The prevalence is thought to be 1% to 10% of the population. Different cultural and ethnic groups may appear avoidant or timid but it may be culturally appropriate, so be careful of these factors when making the diagnosis.

CLINICAL VIGNETTE

Corinne's coworkers at the theater wondered how she could be satisfied working backstage as a prop person for 10 years. Most of them were aspiring actors stuck in the box office or behind the scenes, when they longed to be on stage. Once, as she crossed the stage to place a teapot on a table, Corinne had been caught in the bright lights, and she had nearly fainted. She had gotten her job through her father right after she graduated high school. Although she tried college for a few months, her fear of classmates and missing assignments made her drop out. When a new stage manager with good looks and polite manners was hired at the theater, Corinne tried hard to avoid him. The other women flirted with him. He seemed to like Corinne and wanted to talk to her. Every day she thought about him, but decided she was too ugly to approach him. When she had finally bolstered her confidence to speak with him, she dropped a small radio that she was supposed to place on stage. It seemed to her that the stage manager scowled at her. After that she could not force herself to go near him again.

DISCUSSION

People with APD fear rejection to such an extent that they choose to be lonely rather than risk involvement. Corinne's job as a prop person is perfect for someone with APD. She can stay behind the scenes and easily avoid contact with others. Corinne was fearful and isolated as a child, and during adolescence she stayed away from her peers. She was unable to finish college because of her disorder. Many times, people with APD marry and have children, but they have to be protected and supported by loved ones.

Treatment for APD can consist of individual or group therapy. In individual psychotherapy, the therapist must develop a solid alliance with the patient, maintaining an accepting attitude. As you can see in Corinne's case, the slightest scowl may be misinterpreted as criticism and rejection. She did not have therapy. Her mother encouraged her to date, but Corinne's reluctance could not be overcome.

✦ KEY POINT

Patients with APD must learn to tolerate a world that they perceive as humiliating and rejecting.

Group therapy, if APD patients can be persuaded to commit to being with that many people at once, will help APD patients understand how they are really viewed by other people. At first, they will not believe when people tell them they are OK and not inferior. If they can stay in the group long enough and believe what they are hearing, they may be encouraged to regard the world as a friendlier place that they can enter into.

Medications often used to treat APD include SSRIs, β-blockers, and benzodiazepines. β-blockers decrease autonomic hyperactivity and benzodiazepines modulate GABA receptors, which may be abnormal in APD patients.

9 ▼ Dependent Personality Disorder

> **Essential Concepts**
> - Your Dependent Personality Disorder (DPD) patient will find it hard to make decisions by herself/himself.
> - DPD patients want your support and guidance, because they feel they cannot take care of themselves.
> - They will be afraid to disagree with others or fear doing things on their own.
> - They fear being left alone to care for themselves, and urgently seek a relationship.

> They feel lost when alone because they feel that they cannot do anything without help.
>
> —E. Fromm

People with Dependent Personality Disorder (DPD) rely on others excessively. Even though they may be intelligent and talented, DPD patients have no self-esteem so they wind up clinging to a strong person in their environment. They appear submissive and passive. They may tolerate abusive behavior so that they will be able to maintain connections with their significant others. "Caregivers" will tell the DPD what shirt to wear, who to associate with, what school to attend. If a DPD patient has mental retardation or dementia such dependent behavior is understandable, but when the person is of normal or superior intelligence their reliance on others may be difficult to understand. Often DPD patients are pessimistic and reproachful of themselves, while projecting optimism and all positive virtues on their "caretakers."

KEY POINT

DPD patients will go to extremes to continue to be attached to others.

Sometimes, you see these patients doing unethical and immoral things to maintain their relationships. They will not assume responsibility, so if something is done incorrectly they will turn to the people they are dependent on. In treatment, you must strengthen their self-esteem and show them that they are capable of independent actions and decisions. This is difficult, because they constantly negate themselves and elevate others. Something as small as helping them to give themselves permission to decide what to wear or what to eat each day may be a way to bolster their confidence.

CLINICAL VIGNETTE

Ginny was a 36-year-old assistant director of a TV show. After spending some time with her, most people noticed that Ginny could not make everyday decisions without excessive advice from her boss. He was a dynamic, charismatic, 52-year-old executive producer, the opposite of Ginny.

After the death of her mother, Ginny transferred her dependency needs to her boss. Previously, Ginny had allowed her mother to assume such control over her life that she never married or made any decision without her mother's advice. Ginny expected her boss to assume the same role and found she could not function unless she was within hearing distance of her boss who encouraged her behavior. One late evening when they were on a bedroom set together, they fell into a bed and made love. Once they became lovers her boss distanced himself to avoid suspicion. Unfortunately, Ginny felt helpless without her boss' constant presence. She had difficulty performing her job without his close supervision.

DISCUSSION

At this point, Ginny should have consulted a psychotherapist who could have identified her problem as DPD. The concern in therapy would be that Ginny could become as dependent on the therapist as she had been on her mother and then her boss. The therapist would have to constantly foster independence. For instance, if Ginny asked. "But doctor what should I do?" The therapist would have to refer her back to herself with a question like: "What do you think would be the best plan of action?" instead of answering directly. Ginny would doubt her own advice, but with enough encouragement she might be able to build some self-esteem and independence.

Dependent behavior must be considered in the context of a person's age and sociocultural group. For example, if Ginny were a young child or elderly with many disabilities her dependency could be normal. At 36, medically healthy and from a middle-class American family, Ginny's dependency needs were excessive and pathological.

DPD must be differentiated from dependency as a consequence of a mood or panic disorder or as a result of a medical condition. If someone like Ginny fears abandonment, she will try harder and harder to appease the person on whom she's dependent.

Unfortunately, Ginny never sought therapy and was eventually pushed aside by a competitive assistant director. She was demoted with a decrease in salary. Her boss did not continue the relationship and she unconsciously looked for another authority figure on whom to become dependent.

 KEY POINT

DPD develops in those who have been deprived in childhood.

DPD was first described as "the oral character" by psycho-analysts, characterized by dependence, pessimism, passivity, suggestibility, and lack of perseverance. In 1924, Karl Abraham hypothesized that oral characters develop dependence after being overindulged in the sucking phase, but now more recent studies of child development have ruled out that theory. Those who have been deprived as children and not cared for properly feel an excessive need to get care and feel helpless when alone. Their fear is that they will not be able to care for themselves and they will fail as their early caretakers did.

Obsessive-Compulsive Personality Disorder

You can't be too rich or too thin.

—Gloria Vanderbilt

Patients with Obsessive-Compulsive Personality Disorder (OCPD) are known for their orderliness, perfectionism, and need for control. Their preoccupation with details often derails them from work and they cannot complete tasks. Their scrupulousness and inflexibility about ethics get them into trouble with others. People see them as miserly, uptight, and unpleasant. OCPD patients sacrifice spontaneity for control.

 KEY POINT

OCPD patients are not necessarily afflicted with obsessive-compulsive disorder (OCD).

In OCD, patients have either obsessions or compulsions. The OCPD patient may not suffer from either one, he just has a certain style of behavior and thinking. Obsessions are recurrent and persistent thoughts or impulses that the patient cannot push out of his mind. These thoughts cause anxiety. OCD patients try to ignore the obsessions and they recognize that they are productions of their minds, unlike schizophrenics who might believe that the thoughts are coming from somewhere else. Compulsions may also be possible in OCD patients. They are behaviors, e.g., hand washing, ordering, or mental acts like counting. These behaviors and thoughts are designed to decrease anxiety. However, the obsessions and compulsions themselves cause distress and are time-consuming. Of course, these thoughts and behaviors are not caused by drugs or some medical conditions.

There is a greater prevalence of OCPD in men than in women. There is familial transmission. The psychoanalysts believe that OCPD patients do not trust their emotions and have had harsh discipline in their childhoods. Isolation, reaction formation, and rationalization are defenses that compose an OCPD patient's system.

CLINICAL VIGNETTE

Ron was most comfortable at work, where he managed five employees at a big 24-hour chain drugstore. He was scrupulous, exacting, and honest, and he expected the same from his workers. Ron discovered that John, one of his employees, was not only leaving early every Thursday, but also taking home bottles of Tylenol without paying for them. Ron grabbed John's bag as he tried to leave 1 hour before his shift ended. "I thought so," he said, pulling out two unopened bottles of Tylenol. "The inventory showed these were missing. You're fired!"

"Ron, please let me explain. My mom ..." John begged.

"There's no excuse. Report to the main office on Monday for your last paycheck."

John was a 22-year-old high school dropout who lived with his sick mother in a housing project. He burst into tears. "Mom has cancer. She needs these pills for the pain." Other workers and customers gathered around staring at John and Ron. A man stepped up and offered to pay for the Tylenol.

"That's inappropriate, sir," said Ron, handing the customer back his money. John ran out of the store. Another worker pleaded with Ron to take John back. Ron said no and ordered everyone back to work.

Monday, Ron was called into the main office by his supervisor. "I heard what happened with John," she said carefully from behind her big desk. "We feel you should have given him a break."

"What! He was stealing. I stopped him. That's it." Ron was surprised to hear anyone question him. He was always deferential to authority, but since she did not understand he would explain in great detail. His boss stopped him shortly. "We're concerned that you can't complete jobs and you can't meet schedules."

"I'm very careful and precise. I do a good job." Ron sat up straighter.

"You're too inflexible. Many workers have complained about you. I'm sorry, we're putting you on probation."

"Probation? I work more hours than anyone! Work is my highest priority."

"Sorry. That's our decision."

Ron could not believe it. He had found a thief and saved the company money and he was put on probation! It was not logical. He had been dedicated and conscientious for 15 years. He was worried about finding another job at the age of 55. He did not have a wife or children. He had been too preoccupied with work.

DISCUSSION

Ron was technically correct that John should not have been stealing, but Ron needed to be flexible enough to consider John's circumstances and give him another chance. John was a much beloved employee who had grown up in a poor environment. He had resisted crime, but his mother's predicament caused him to act impulsively. Ron was cold and indifferent to him and other workers. He forced his workers to submit and do things exactly his way, which was often not the best way. Ironically, it was Ron who was fired from his job and John kept on. Ron did not feel anger about the injustice, he just ruminated about what things he should take from his desk. He needed to maintain control over his emotions and his environment.

Often patients with OCPD do not visit psychiatrists unless they become depressed or anxious. They must be differentiated from those with Narcissistic Personality Disorder, who believe that they are perfect rather than seeking perfection, and from patients with Antisocial Personality Disorder, who are similarly ungenerous but mistreat people constantly. People with Schizoid Personality Disorder may also be detached and formal, but those with OCPD are more uncomfortable with emotions and dedicated to work.

 KEY POINT

The best way to treat your OCPD patients is to gently interrupt their lists of things.

OCPD patients will respond to you stopping their onslaught of details if you do it gently. Do not criticize their need for perfection, but keep pointing out that they should focus on completion of tasks. They cannot understand delegating work to others or lack of schedules. Therapy should be supportive or insight-oriented. Group therapy may be beneficial.

Personality Disorder, Not Otherwise Specified

Essential Concepts
- Your Personality Disorder Not Otherwise Specified (PDNOS) will not fit nicely into any of the usual categories.
- PDNOS patients meet the general criteria for personality disorders.
- At present, people with Passive-Aggressive Personality Disorder and Depressive Personality Disorder are PDNOS patients.
- PDNOS patients may have a mixture of many personality disorders.

Personality Disorder Not Otherwise Specified (PDNOS) patients were called "mixed personalities" in the past. They have impaired social and occupational functioning.

Passive-Aggressive Personality Disorder, Self-Defeating Personality Disorder, and Depressive Personality Disorder can all be listed as PDNOS patients. If a patient has one particular trait or a behavior that cannot be classified anywhere else, PDNOS can be used.

 KEY POINT

If a patient has borderline, histrionic, and narcissistic features that are all prominent components of his personality, use PDNOS.

Clinicians will often treat patients who cannot easily be tucked into one category or another. Unfortunately, real life does not always conform to our classification system. When the DSMV is published we may have more or less categories of personality disorder, but we will always have PDNOS.

CLINICAL VIGNETTE

Even in early childhood, Ann would sit in her bedroom alone, isolated, and brooding. She thought about dying, because she felt worthless and dejected. Her family was not sure what was bothering her, but they realized that it was better not to call her down to play or eat dinner. If interrupted, she screamed and had tantrums. Ann always surprised her family with her degree of animosity, because her blond braids and blue eyes made her look so friendly and sweet.

Ann's dejection and gloominess continued to dominate her moods as she moved through adolescence into adulthood. In high school, she hung out with the "Goths" and took downer drugs with them. Ann and her friends dressed in black, painted their fingernails red, and powdered their faces dead white. By the time she was 17, Ann had three DWIs. Ann was given Celexa and antidepressants by the school psychiatrist. It did not help. In college, she excelled in her studies despite being drawn to the "dark side." A boyfriend introduced her to painkillers. She wound up using as many as a dozen per day. When she was high, she no longer had to deal with her unhappiness. She just "spaced out" in front of the TV. Ann always complained about feeling "empty inside" anyway. One night she took an overdose of Vicodin and had to be brought to the emergency room and then admitted to the psychiatric ward.

DISCUSSION

Ann can be categorized as having a Depressive Personality Disorder because her usual mood is dejection, gloomy, and cheerless. She feels inadequate and worthless and is critical of herself as well as pessimistic. She also has many characteristics of a Borderline Personality Disorder patient with feelings of emptiness, substance abuse, and irritability. In addition, she can be considered narcissistic.

A patient like Ann would best be described as a PDNOS. Depressive Personality Disorder is considered a criteria set that needs further research. The best plan to combat her drug addiction and suicidal behavior is to hospitalize her and use a 12-step program for treatment.

 KEY POINT

You can treat the drug problem, but do not expect to alleviate PDNOS.

A patient like Ann will benefit from her hospitalization and follow up in AA or NA, but the clinician should not expect to improve her mood or change her self-concept or increase her self-esteem very much. Remember that personality disorders are notoriously intransigent by their nature.

12 Schizotypal Personality Disorder

He was such a strange man, he sent shivers down my spine.

> —A nurse on an inpatient unit in Bellevue Hospital Center in New York City

Schizotypal Personality Disorder (SPD) must be contrasted with Schizoid Personality Disorder (see Chapter 3) because the two are so often confused. SPD patients are extremely uncomfortable in social relationships, but they are different from patients with Schizoid Personality Disorder, who are also unable to engage in normal social interactions comfortably, in that they are strange and paranoid. Schizoid Personality Disorder patients are not as weird; they are just isolated. SPD patients may be superstitious or interested in the paranormal. Other people perceive them as eccentric and different, whereas the public does not think of Schizoid Personality Disorder people in this way. Another difference between Schizoid and Schizotypal Personality Disorder is that SPD patients want to have relationships, whereas Schizoid Personality Disorder people do not. SPD patients have trouble with relationships because of their ideas of reference, odd beliefs and speech, anxiety, and paranoia. SPD patients cannot trust others in a relationship.

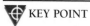 KEY POINT

The social phobia your patient is experiencing may be an Axis II Personality Disorder.

Many times we simply believe that a patient is suffering from social phobia, but if we take a thorough history and review of symptoms we understand that a personality disorder may underlie the problems, especially if the patient is particularly strange and paranoid. If there is difficulty in engaging a patient and he is eccentric with a constricted affect, yet he is not floridly psychotic with hallucinations and delusions, then he very well may have SPD. People with social phobia are afraid of social or performance situations and fear that they will humiliate themselves. They know their fears are excessive and they avoid exposure. However, they are not odd or paranoid.

Patients with SPD symptoms can also have schizophrenia. In earlier versions of the DSM, decisions were made to separate SPD and other Cluster A diagnoses from schizophrenia in the hopes that a spectrum of disorders would be helpful in considering clinical and familial aspects of treatment.

CLINICAL VIGNETTE

George was a handsome 25-year-old, who dressed in dark, loose clothing that made him appear odd rather than fashionable. He complained about his fear of people. His stiff body movements and wide-brimmed hats, which he pulled down to avoid eye contact, alienated him from others. He visited a psychiatrist for his social phobia and had Lexapro 10 mg prescribed. After 1 month, he reported feeling less embarrassed and awkward around coworkers. As a member of the IT staff of a giant company, he had to go from desk to desk, computer to computer, and teach colleagues how to use programs he designed. He was afraid that his hands would shake during these interactions. George's father, an alcoholic, had beaten and terrorized him as a young boy. His mother was also tough and demanding, expecting perfection from him. In childhood, George had isolated himself in his room and worked on his computer. He excelled in schoolwork and skateboarding. Lexapro helped him feel a little more comfortable around coworkers, but then he revealed that on the subway, he had to position himself in such a way that he did not invade other people's "energy" fields and that they did not invade his. This meant sitting with his legs together, head down, and hands in his lap. If he deviated from this posture, he believed men would be hostile and women would send out "sexual vibrations." With this revelation, the psychiatrist added Abilify 5 mg to his regime. A week later the patient reported feeling better.

DISCUSSION

It could be argued that there was some reality to his concerns on the subway. If he spread his legs far apart, other riders on the crowded train might consider him territorial and invasive of space or women might notice him and flirt. However, George's ideas of reference, magical thinking, and paranoia placed him into the category of SPD. His ability to feel better around his coworkers after medication and the fact that he was able to relax somewhat on the subway did not disqualify him from the SPD criteria. Many times medications can be helpful to personality disorder patients, but they are never "cured." SPD must be distinguished from delusional disorder, schizophrenia, and mood disorder with psychotic features.

 KEY POINT

Try not to be judgmental of patients, if they believe in the occult or other strange things.

SPD patients beliefs tend to run to the mystical or occult. During psychotherapy, the therapist may be too eager to set SPD patients straight. Avoid being directive about magical thinking, because this attitude may be more productive in promoting an alliance with your patient. Tolerance of SPD patients' oddness will be of great help to them.

13

Passive-Aggressive
Personality Disorder

Essential Points
- Your Passive-Aggressive Personality Disorder (PAPD) patients will be sullen and resentful.
- They will passively resist doing their work or social obligations.
- They feel misunderstood, envious, and resentful.
- They criticize and scorn authority and defy it.

Why should I do any work?
—A patient with Passive-Aggressive
Personality Disorder

The person with PAPD is negative and passive in the workplace and in his social circle. Other people find that they have to struggle to interact with him. He feels hostile unconsciously, which he cannot express directly, so he passively resists interactions. PAPD patients procrastinate, resist, give excuses, and generally derail any attempts toward progress. They cannot directly say what they need or want. People experience them as punishing and manipulative, but they might just be dependent and self-detrimental. PAPD patients resent and feel misunderstood by most people. The treating clinician must be patient and try to understand their negative point of view. Then after an alliance is formed, if it is, the clinician can point out how angry the patient actually is. PAPD patients can be encouraged to express their anger directly. This is very difficult for them. As children they were punished for expressing anger directly, but it is exactly what they need to do. If the clinician just fulfills their demands the patients learn nothing. Nevertheless, if their demands are refused, then PAPD patients will feel rejected, sending them spiraling down into resentment. A fine balance must be drawn with them. Therapists should be supportive, but not coddling.

 KEY POINT

PAPD patients have opposite and conflicting needs, one for dependence and the other for independence.

As a result of this struggle for dependence on another person coupled with the need for independence, the PAPD winds up frozen in action. Long ago, the PAPD patient learned to squelch his anger and active needs. To unlock active aggression is not easy when the patient has spent years bottling it up. Opposition to authority is a typical symptom in PAPD and may be accompanied by envy and resentment of peers who have no problems with authority. PAPD patients are constantly disappointed and arguing.

CLINICAL VIGNETTE

Jan had been working as a postal clerk for 25 years. Whenever she felt inadequate she would tell herself that she really was destined for more prestigious work, but that she was a victim of circumstances, having been born to a single, impoverished, and abusive mother who stopped Jan from finishing high school. At the post office, customers complained that Jan was the slowest, meanest clerk on the floor. No matter how many times supervisors reprimanded her, Jan dawdled. She knew she was in no danger of losing her job. Jan felt angry since the customers were so demanding all day long. Instead of expressing this directly or trying to help herself in any way, she passively resisted routine tasks. When someone approached her post office window, she would purposely ignore them for several minutes as she straightened papers and sipped coffee.

When she finally accepted the customer's package or letter, she grabbed it, threw it on the scale, and scowled. Jan liked making people squirm. When coworkers asked her for help Jan was sullen or argumentative, alternating between hostile defiance and contrition. Often she would delay her appearance at a coworker's window or misplace needed documents. Jan was quick to criticize authority and voice resentment at those she perceived as more fortunate than herself.

DISCUSSION

Jan clearly had PAPD. Her negative attitudes and passive resistance to demands for performance were detrimental to herself and her workplace. Jan felt powerless so she acted out passively.

Few PAPD patients present themselves for treatment. Instead, they are busy acting out by procrastinating, complaining, resisting, and resenting. In Jan's case, she finally ventured into treatment to help her son who was in a drug rehab for crack smoking. He promised his mother he would stay sober if she would be supportive. Jan felt manipulated. Her son's therapist encouraged them to go on an NA meeting together. Jan went and while there the counselor encouraged Jan to express her anger at her son's drug use. Usually, she could not but suddenly she surprised herself by exploding with rage. Sometimes, PAPD patients can rise to an occasion and become appropriately angry, especially to help family members.

KEY POINT

PAPD patients will blame others for failure and chronically complain.

They externalize blame and have difficulty taking responsibility. Authority figures are easy scapegoats for them. They complain about personal misfortune and imagine that other people have it so much better than they do. They are ambivalent. They may have a superficial bravado, but all is chaos internally. As they are such defeatists, other people will be negative and hostile toward them.

In childhood, they may have Oppositional Defiant Disorder. PAPD is diagnosed in adults when the personality traits have become inflexible and maladaptive. PAPD is considered a Personality Disorder Not Otherwise Specified (PDNOS) at this point.

Antidepressants can be prescribed when they have major depression. Of course, these medications will not break down the patterns of negative thinking, but cognitive behavioral therapy may be useful for them.

Self-Defeating Personality Disorder

Sometimes love don't feel like it should. You make it hurt it so good.

—"Hurts So Good," John Mellencamp

The superego is exaggerated in the Self-Defeating Personality Disorder (SdPD) patient, whereas the ego is diminished. As a consequence, patients need to punish themselves over and over again. We call this condition moral masochism. It is not listed in DSM-IV-TR, but it is well known in psychiatry. Sexual masochism is listed. Many times, patients with SdPD will engage in physical and sexual acts to hurt themselves. Underneath, patients have a strong sense of guilt. Frustrating themselves satisfies that guilt.

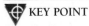 KEY POINT

Sadistic aspects are present, but they are mostly repressed.

Usually, elements of both masochistic and sadistic behaviors are present in the same person. Sadism and masochism represent two opposite extremes of the subjugation—humiliation spectrum. Both are related to the fear of injury and a reactive narcissistic rage. If SdPD patients engage in psychotherapy, they must be made aware of their needs for self-punishment secondary to excessive unconscious guilt. It is also necessary for these patients to recognize repressed, aggressive impulses that originate in childhood.

CLINICAL VIGNETTE

Roberta, a graduate student in psychology, was interested in all aspects of human behavior. Yet her own actions were often a mystery to her. She struggled throughout her undergrad studies and finally at 29, won a full scholarship to a prestigious university. Ostensibly, she was happy to be starting her life's work. However, she could not bring herself to attend classes or do any of the assignments. Her favorite professor, who had recommended Roberta for the scholarship and mentored her, demanded an explanation. Roberta could provide no honest excuse. As much as she liked the professor and the classes, she had only attended three times during the entire semester. When the time came to hand in the term paper, Roberta had another problem. Her topic was clear to her, her preparation ample, but she wound up turning the paper in at the last minute. Her favorite professor placed Roberta on probation. Roberta was not surprised, throughout her school years she had been in trouble many times for the same problem. As bright and talented as she was she also had been expelled from two schools in the past. It was not simply a matter of procrastination. Roberta also defeated herself in social relationships. Instead of dating men her own age, she chose men who were too young or too old. Roberta laughed at herself and encouraged others to mock her as well. She enjoyed the negative attention if others made her the butt of a joke. On one date, she engaged in painful sex and found that she enjoyed it. Hoping to gain some insight, Roberta consulted a psychiatrist at the university's health center. At the beginning of treatment, Roberta would either miss the session completely or show up for the last 10 minutes. The psychiatrist patiently explained this behavior to Roberta as avoidance. She understood and armed with this knowledge she was able to change her pattern and attend more sessions. She also went to classes more frequently.

DISCUSSION

The psychiatrist pointed out that Roberta's punitive mother could not be pleased by anything she did. Roberta responded by forming a harsh superego that was eager to inflict punishment on herself. Her guilt made her defeat herself constantly. Instead of allowing herself to achieve gratification and increase self-esteem by attending classes, writing papers, or finding an appropriate mate, Roberta frustrated herself at every step. She satisfied her superego and defeated her ego; in other words, she was a moral masochist, but sexual masochism drove her into treatment.

In DSM-III-R, SdPD was a proposed diagnostic category needing further study. After debate, the category was removed from DSM-IV completely. It is not clear whether or not it will be included in DSM-V.

 KEY POINT

The SdPD will respond with depression or guilt to new achievements.

Remember they always want to defeat themselves.

AXIS I
INTERSECTING
AXIS II

Personality Disorders and Major Depression

> **Essential Concepts**
> - Any patient with a personality disorder can also have major depression.
> - The symptoms of depression will manifest differently through the prism of the personality disorder.
> - Some personality disorder patients will seem to be depressed all the time but they really are not.
> - The medications that we use may be the same for depression no matter what personality disorder, but the psychotherapy will differ.

Trailed by the black dog of depression.

—Winston Churchill

Why did the authors of the DSM divide disorders into Axis I and Axis II? They wanted to make sure that we understood that whatever the clinical disorder (Axis I) was, any personality disorder (Axis II) would affect the course and outcome tremendously. There is a lot of controversy about personality disorders with clinicians trying to squeeze various patients into the given personality disorder categories. Some say there is inadequate scientific basis for the criteria. Others complain that there are arbitrary boundaries between normal personalities and abnormal ones. People sharing categories may be completely different from one another. Whatever the complaints, most of us find the Axis II diagnoses very useful when dealing with difficult patients. The problems arise when patients get penalized by insurance reimbursements or other doctors by the labels we impart.

Major Depression is one of the most common Axis I psychiatric diagnosis, yet it is estimated that only about 20% of those with depression seek treatment. Certain personality disorder patients like those with Dependent Personality Disorder and Borderline Personality Disorder may seek treatment more than the average person. Those with Paranoid, Schizoid, or Avoidant Personality Disorder may seek treatment less often.

 KEY POINT

A person has major depression if he/she has at least five of the following symptoms nearly every day for two weeks: insomnia or hypersomnia; overeating; undereating; feeling of sadness; thoughts of suicide; irritability; guilt; low self-esteem; decreased concentration; loss of interest in sex and other activities; restlessness or fatigue.

A Paranoid Personality Disorder patient may be even more hostile and withdrawn when he has depression. He will not cry in public and will probably hide suicidal thoughts and other weaknesses. Therefore, be especially careful to assess for suicidal intentions.

A schizoid personality will become more anhedonic and withdrawn. He or she will not be able to feel the sadness fully, but they may be more fatigued. Dig for the other symptoms of depression.

Schizotypals may become more anxious and their belief systems can get stranger. Be sure they do not have psychotic depression with hallucinations or delusions.

Antisocial personalities may be more impulsive, aggressive, and irritable. You may notice that their criminal behavior increases.

Borderline personalities fight with others more. Their anger may be overwhelming. Their self-damaging acts increase. Look out for suicidal threats and actions.

Histrionic personalities cry and seek your attention and concern. They won't look as good as usual, because they won't have the capacity to care for themselves while depressed.

Narcissistic personality disorders may be even more arrogant and exploitative. They will be even more entitled than usual. Crying will occur if they feel it will get them more of a "special" status.

Avoidants will feel more inadequate and withdrawn with poor self-images. Do worry about them committing suicide. Dependents, on the other hand, will lean heavily on their significant relationships and seek the most nurturance they can.

Obsessive-Compulsive personalities will be very hard on themselves and everyone else. They rigidly and stubbornly try to stick to their usual rituals, but they will not be able to.

CLINICAL VIGNETTE

Ray, a 59-year-old dance teacher, always thought of herself as beautiful and "special." She had been on the stage in more than a few musicals. Her favorite stories were ones about how "gorgeous" she looked in her costumes and how men admired her long legs. For years after the stage, she had obtained her admiration and sense of entitlement from her husband. Unfortunately, when he began to suffer from Alzheimer's disease. Ray had to spend most of her time indoors, taking care of him. She decided to retire early since she was constantly exhausted and unable to keep up with her energetic students. Ray believed she was perfectly fine, if only she could get some rest. Her disturbed sleep was blamed exclusively on her husband, who slept in the same bed and woke at least four times each night to wander. Ray would wake too and follow him around the apartment to make sure he was safe. When her son called, he would find her crying or too lethargic to speak. Her appetite diminished. Her internist found her in fine physical shape when she went for a checkup. Her constant zest for life was gone. One day she surprised everyone by announcing that she wished she had died in a car accident she had survived many years before. Her son suspected she was depressed and urged her to get treatment. She insisted that her depression was due to her husband's condition. After much discussion, Ray visited a psychopharmacologist, who obtained a thorough history and found out this was Ray's third untreated episode of major depression. He prescribed 10 mg of Lexapro. After four weeks, Ray regained her appetite, slept well, regained her vigor for life, and was "ready to dance." Her usually rational perspective on difficult matters returned and she hired a nurse's aide for her husband. Of course, her "specialness," need for admiration, sense of entitlement, and haughtiness remained the same.

 KEY POINT

You can treat the Axis I condition but do not expect to cure the Axis II diagnoses.

DISCUSSION

Ray failed to obtain what she needed from her husband once he became demented. This caused depression, but it may not have been major depression. In Ray's case it was. She met all the criteria, but she was in denial about it. Most people believe that if they are coping with a tragic event they have a right to be depressed. They think their depression will be relieved as soon as the tragedy is alleviated or that the depression is dependent on the event. This is untrue; if the depression is ongoing for six months, then the person's brain chemistry has changed and she may be clinically depressed. Ray's vegetative signs, i.e., decreased appetite, insomnia, and fatigue, were sure indications of her condition.

If left untreated, depression may lead to suicide. Depression is very treatable with medication. We have a wealth of antidepressants from SSRIs to TCAs to MAOIs. New medications are being developed constantly. CBT and other forms of psychotherapy may be used as well. ECT is also an effective treatment.

Depressed people are likely to negatively influence their homes and workplaces. They are apt to lose jobs, alienate friends and family, because untreated, depressed people are often seen as lazy, ineffective, and difficult. Therefore, patients who have both a personality disorder and major depression are in twice as much trouble as anyone else. Suicide and miserable lives may be a result of untreated depression, so the clinician must be alert to the very treatable condition of depression.

16

Personality Disorders and Bipolar Disorder

> **Essential Points**
> - The most common types of personality disorders found coinciding with Bipolar Disorder are Borderline Personality Disorder and Narcissistic Personality Disorder.
> - The personality disorder may be masked if the patient is a rapid cycler.
> - Schizotypal Personality Disorder should be considered if the bipolar patient returns to an abnormal state after mania or hypomania.
> - Depressions can be treated with medications as well as manic episodes, but do not expect to affect the underlying personality disorder.

> Scratch a bipolar patient, get a borderline underneath.
>
> —Unknown

Many clinicians are familiar with the hostility of patients suffering from both Borderline Personality Disorder and Bipolar Disorder. When a bipolar I patient is in a manic state or even in a hypomanic state, he may be physically and emotionally aggressive toward others or even toward himself, in the form of suicidal behavior. The patient with Borderline Personality Disorder may present with a similar hostility and/or aggression. If your bipolar patient is not hypomanic or manic and he still is angry at everyone including himself, it may be that he also has Borderline Personality Disorder. If your bipolar patient is full of a sense of his own importance and requires excessive admiration, then the underlying condition may very well be Narcissistic Personality Disorder.

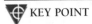 **KEY POINT**

For a diagnosis of bipolar disorder, your patient must have elevated moods alternating with depression.

People are often confused about unipolar depression versus bipolar depression. Major depression is present if a patient has five or more of these symptoms for a two-week period: (1) depressed mood (sad), (2) decreased interest or pleasure in usual activities, (3) weight loss or gain, (4) insomnia or hypersomnia, (5) agitation or retardation, (6) fatigue or loss of energy, (7) feelings of worthlessness or inappropriate guilt, (8) decreased concentration, and (9) suicidal ideation. If in addition to periods of depression your patient also has manic episodes, which are inflated self-esteem, decreased sleep, pressured speech, racing thoughts, distractibility, and foolish behavior, then you have a bipolar I patient. Sometimes, bipolar I patients can also have delusions and hallucinations during a manic episode. Bipolar II patients have hypomanic episodes, which are elevated expansive or irritable moods that last 4 days accompanied by inflated self-esteem, decreased sleep, and flight of ideas. Bipolar II patients do not hallucinate and are not delusional. If your patient has delusions and/or hallucinations, he or she must have the bipolar I diagnosis.

When you add an Axis II diagnosis to major depression and/or bipolar disorder, things get complicated. A Paranoid Personality Disorder patient may cycle into persecutory delusions and hallucinate if he also has bipolar I disorder. A Borderline Personality Disorder patient may be particularly irritable at times when he cycles into a hypomanic episode and he has a bipolar II diagnosis as well.

CLINICAL VIGNETTE

Jack, a 30-year-old high school English teacher, had emotional ups and downs throughout his life. Last winter, he was so depressed that he considered throwing himself off the terrace of his high-rise apartment to stop his torment. He gained 20 pounds and found himself sleeping 12 hours per night. His depression remitted in March, but approximately a month later, strange things started happening. Jack, who was sober for 2 years, found himself filled with unusual energy that reminded him of what it felt like when he was drinking every day. At school, Jack's coworkers commented on his high energy level. His students complained that he went through material so quickly that there was no time to take notes. When they asked questions, Jack, ordinarily patient, snapped at them. His bursts of creative energy reminded him of his adolescence. One night he sat down and wrote two short stories and a poem. On the spur of the moment, Jack took a trip to Atlantic City and spent more money in 5 hours of gambling than he had in years. He had sex with three different prostitutes. When he returned to New York City, he was still overexcited and he jumped into the lake in Central Park. He said he wanted to see whether he could swim across. The police came and rescued him from the freezing water. At the local emergency room, a psychiatrist on call tentatively diagnosed him with bipolar I disorder. Jack was given Risperdal and Li_2CO_3. He responded well to the medications and only missed a few days of work during his entire manic episode.

When he returned to his normal state, he still felt "special" and needed admiration from his coworkers and students. He was as grandiose as ever, feeling he was "as good a writer as Hemingway." He still lacked empathy and he was arrogant about his good looks and abilities. Jack's Narcissistic Personality Disorder was not affected by Risperdal and Li_2CO_3, although his bipolar I disorder was under control.

DISCUSSION

Jack's depressive winter episode is typical of many bipolars. In this pattern known as seasonal affective disorder (SAD), individuals become melancholic in the winter and then experience mania in the spring. Before Jack had a full-blown manic or depressive period, he had cyclothymia, i.e., he "cycled" back and forth between depression and mania each year at the appropriate season. Jack's age of onset, 30, is common for bipolar disorder. During a manic episode, individuals move and talk quickly. Many bipolar patients find that some of their most innovative ideas occur during manic episodes. If they are able to harness this energy and apply it to work situations, they can function well. The problem is that many of these ideas are lost when the individual returns to normal. Many patients on lithium claim that this medication decreases their creativity, and so they stop the medication prematurely.

Judgment is adversely affected in bipolar disorder. Jack lost a large amount of money gambling, had unprotected sex with high-risk partners, and jumped into a freezing lake during his manic episode. His history of alcoholism is also common among patients with bipolar disorder as is concurrent alcoholism or drug abuse. Jack's problems were decreased, and his diagnosis facilitated by the fact that he was sober. Risperdal was stopped after three weeks and Jack did well on lithium maintenance. He still found himself cycling up and down with the seasons (and of course he still had Narcissistic Personality Disorder), but he did not have any more manic or depressive episodes. Jack was extremely fortunate; not all patients do as well. Many continue to have manic and depressive episodes even with lithium. Many patients need other mood stabilizers such as Depakote, Tegretol, Neurontin, and Lamictal to remain in remission.

Bipolar disorder is not as debilitating as schizophrenia. Even if a person has a manic or psychotic episode, he or she usually returns to the premorbid state intact. However, when the bipolar patient also has Narcissistic Personality Disorder, he may not share all his problems with his doctor because he wants to present an idealized version of himself to you. Therefore, with a patient like Jack, it is important to bring in other people in the family, if there is anyone, to collaborate information.

If Jack had not returned to a normal state after mania, then Schizotypal Personality Disorder would have to be ruled out. For instance, if Jack had odd beliefs about his abilities or magical thinking about himself and he was not as personable, then a diagnosis of Schizotypal Personality Disorder may have been made.

In a rapidly cycling patient, the extremes of depression and mania or hypomania are occurring so quickly, many diagnoses may be masked. Remember most depressions look unipolar at first. Bipolar disorder is often not considered, so antidepressants are freely prescribed, especially by clinicians who are not psychiatrists. Then when the bipolar patient cycles into a manic episode, a psychiatrist is called in. Antidepressants are necessary when a bipolar patient is depressed, but they must be used with caution and many times with the addition of mood stabilizers and/or antipsychotics. A psychiatrist will examine the patient's history in great detail and try to determine whether it is just unipolar or whether it is bipolar disorder. Patterns of eating, sleeping, energy, and mood will be scrutinized. Sometimes, it is not possible to determine whether the patient is bipolar on the first visit.

17 Personality Disorders and Panic Attacks

Essential Concepts
- Any patient with a personality disorder may also have panic attacks.
- The most common types of personality disorder found with panic disorder are Dependent Personality Disorder and Avoidant Personality Disorder.
- Panic disorder is easily treatable; personality disorders are not.
- Untreated panic attack patients can go on to develop agoraphobia and Avoidant Personality Disorder.

Panic disorder is quite common with a lifetime prevalence rate of 1.5% to 3.5%. Anxiety disorders themselves are among the most frequently occurring psychiatric problems in the general population. A panic attack is a certain period of intense fear or discomfort that comes upon an individual out of nowhere, for no particular reason. Panic attacks are not triggered by internal or external stimuli the way simple phobia is. Later in the course of the disorder, panic attacks may be triggered by a situation in which a patient previously had a panic attack.

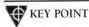 KEY POINT

If the patient is always panicked about a certain situation or event, it probably is an anxiety attack, not a panic attack.

Panic attacks reach a peak in 10 minutes and include four or more of the following symptoms: palpitations, pounding heart or increased heart rate, sweating, trembling, shortness of breath, choking feeling, chest pain, nausea, dizziness, derealization or depersonalization, fear of losing control, fear of dying, paresthesias, and chills or hot flashes.

Patients are often taken to the emergency room (ER) because they believe they are having a heart attack. Once they know they are having panic attacks, they can seek treatment with a psychiatrist. For the diagnosis of panic disorder, the patient needs to have recurrent, *unexpected* panic attacks, and then at least one month of concern about having panic attacks. If the patient is not worried about panic attacks, then it is probably not panic disorder, but various personality disorders affect the way patients express fears. For instance, if we are dealing with a Paranoid Personality Disorder patient, he may not want to share the fact that he is having panic attacks, because he is afraid that this information can be used against him. A Borderline Personality Disorder patient may use her panic attacks to be angry at the injustice of the world. A histrionic one may exaggerate the panic attack so that she can get the most attention from the medical staff attending her, whereas the Schizoid Personality Disorder patient may draw further into himself when having a panic attack.

Dependent Personality Disorder patients will use the panic attacks as proof that they should never be left alone, and should always be cared for by others. Avoidant Personality Disorder patients will have the perfect excuse to stay away from other people and situations. They will constantly fear that a panic attack will occur, so they will not try to go anywhere or accomplish anything. It is necessary to identify and treat panic attacks with these patients as soon as possible, so that they do not develop agoraphobia, which is the fear of going outside.

Most people with panic disorder are affected in their twenties: most are women. One theory has it that panic attacks are caused by a falsely activated alarm system in the brain, an area called the locus ceruleus. The major concentration of adrenergic neurons is located there. Axons of these nerve cells are connected into the cerebral cortex, the limbic system, the thalamus, and the hypothalamus. The patient has noradrenergic overload when the false alarm goes off. Panic attack patients are flooded with adrenaline, which makes them feel frightened and triggers a "fight or flight" response when nothing bad is actually happening in their environment. Early human beings developed these systems to defend themselves from enemies and escape danger. Like any alarm systems, they can easily go astray. Data are showing that panic attacks are also caused by abnormalities in GABA or serotonin systems in the brain. Clearly, panic attacks are caused by chemical imbalances in the nervous system and not by a patient's imagination, as many people might claim. Antidepressants, which are used to treat panic attacks (more on that in Section III), downregulate neuroreceptors in the locus ceruleus. Downregulation of receptors may be a healing process of the faulty alarm system. In about 50% of cases, treatment of panic attacks with antidepressants for one year will lead to a panic-attack-free life afterward.

CLINICAL VIGNETTE

Penny, a 23-year-old police officer, was proud to have a job that was somewhat unusual for women. Ever since she was nine, and had watched her father in his police uniform, she had wanted to join the force. She did well in basic training and always volunteered for jobs and territories that most of her coworkers disliked.

Penny always believed she was "special" and she needed the admiration of her parents, her partners, and her friends. When alone, she fantasized about rescuing celebrities from their fans and achieving world recognition.

One day a dreadful thing happened to Penny that completely changed her life. She was riding the passenger seat in the patrol car with her partner on their way to apprehend a shoplifter. Suddenly, Penny felt as if she were thrown forward. She clutched at the dashboard frantically as her heart pounded and her body trembled. Nausea, dizziness, and breathlessness hit her hard. Worst of all, she felt as if she were outside herself, watching herself die. Her partner pulled over to the curb and tried to help her. He could not calm her, so he drove her to the ER for care. There they drew blood tests and did an EKG. All was normal. Penny went to an internist the next day. Again, he found everything to be normal. She was told to take it easy and stop working so hard. Penny did not feel that her job was taxing. She went back to working as hard as ever. The second week after the first incident, she had another attack, two days later she had a third. All of them occurred outdoors, so Penny associated being outside with the attacks. There was no way to predict when one would occur. She was constantly nervous and worried that she would have an attack in a situation that demanded her full wits or strength. Waiting for an attack was almost as bad as having one. Where Penny was once carefree and cheerful, she became worried and morose. The attacks were a narcissistic injury to her self-esteem. After she had a panic attack in the subway while arresting two muggers, who almost escaped due to her distraction, Penny was assigned to a desk job. Her constant anticipation of panic attacks made her irritable and difficult. Coworkers tiptoed around her. Eventually, Penny needed her boyfriend to take her to work and bring her home at the end of the day. Penny had wanted to be a police officer to show herself and her family that women could be independent and courageous. She was disgusted that she became so dependent. Penny suffered for two years like this until she saw an advertisement for an anxiety clinic and consulted a psychiatrist. Her disorder was easily diagnosed as panic disorder. She was given 25 mg Zoloft and instructed to slowly increase the dose to 100 mg over several days. After three weeks on 100 mg, Penny was relieved of panic attacks. She could not believe she had endured them for two years. Penny had to re-expand her life and work. She was reassigned to field work. It felt good to ride around in the patrol car once again and not worry about impending panic attacks. She no longer needed her boyfriend to accompany her to and from work. Penny was pleasantly surprised to regain all of her previous functions.

DISCUSSION

Penny's case of panic disorder is not unusual. Many panic patients are brought to an ER under the misconception that they are having a heart attack. After the standard physical problems are ruled out, panic disorder must be considered. For Penny, two years of misery and decreased work efficacy could have been avoided if a panic disorder diagnosis could have been considered initially.

Many untreated panic attack patients go on to develop agoraphobia. This avoidance behavior leads to travel and location restrictions. An individual with agoraphobia may need companionship every time she travels. Common situations that become difficult or impossible for agoraphobics to manage include being outside alone; in a crowd or line; going over bridges; and traveling in a bus, train, or car. Some agoraphobics become housebound.

Penny's Narcissistic Personality Disorder was in the background while her panic disorder was prominent. She felt "special" from the panic attacks, but "injured" by her inability to perform as she once had. She was driven further into her fantasies of rescuing people as she sat bored at her desk job. When she was finally relieved of her panic attacks she returned to her arrogance and entitlement, whereas a patient without Narcissistic Personality Disorder might have learned to be more humble and grateful for her return of health.

Panic disorder can recur when treatment is discontinued. About 30% to 90% of successfully treated panic disorder patients relapse. Penny should be careful about discontinuing her medications. She should have follow-up sessions with a psychiatrist at least a few times per year.

Personality Disorders and Schizophrenia

Essential Concepts

- A patient may have schizophrenia and any personality disorder, except probably not Paranoid, Schizotypal, or Schizoid Personality Disorder.
- A schizophrenic patient may premorbidly be diagnosed with Schizotypal or Paranoid or Schizoid Personality Disorder.
- The most common types of personality disorders seen with schizophrenia are Obsessive-Compulsive and Borderline Personality Disorders.
- If a patient is experiencing delusions and/or hallucinations for one month or longer, it is most probably schizophrenia and not just a personality disorder.

The term (schizophrenia) is widely misunderstood, especially by the lay public, as signifying a split personality.

—Kaplan and Sadock's *Synopsis of Psychiatry*

Symptoms of schizophrenia are usually categorized into negative or positive ones. Positive symptoms include delusions, hallucinations, disorganized speech, and behavior. Negative symptoms are restrictions in range and intensity of emotions, affective flattering, alogia, and avolition.

In 1930, Bleuler described the four A's of schizophrenia, which are still useful to us. (1) Association—i.e., looseness of associations; (2) Affect—inappropriate and flat emotional states; (3) Autism—self-involved, turned away from the world; (4) Ambivalence—the patient has difficulty making up his mind and swings back and forth between the negative and positive sides of issues.

For paranoid, schizoid, and schizotypal personality disorders, DSM-IV-TR provides exclusion criteria, stating that the pattern of behavior must not have occurred exclusively during the course of schizophrenia, a mood disorder with psychotic features or another psychotic disorder. If a patient has a chronic Axis I condition like schizophrenia that was preceded by a pre-existing personality disorder, then the personality disorder should be marked as "premorbid." It is probably less confusing with schizophrenic patients not to consider paranoid, schizoid, or schizotypal personality disorders in their Axis II diagnoses.

 KEY POINT

Schizotypal, Paranoid, and Borderline Personality Disorder patients can all have delusions, but they do not have hallucinations like schizophrenics.

If your patient is having auditory or visual hallucinations, then you should consider schizophrenia as a diagnosis, even if your patient just started with some paranoid delusions and you thought that you were just dealing with a Paranoid Personality Disorder or a Schizotypal Personality Disorder or a Borderline Personality Disorder. Once the realm of psychosis is entered by the patient having frank hallucinations, a mere diagnosis of a personality disorder may be inadequate. Of course, you may also be dealing with a bipolar I disorder or a temporary psychosis or a substance-induced disorder.

 KEY POINT

Stress can often bring out an Axis I condition in patients with Axis II personality disorders.

CLINICAL VIGNETTE

Sara, at 22, did not mind that people could not distinguish her from five other bank clerks who worked beside her. She did not complain when customers ignored her or called her by the wrong name. Her humility was not a sign of good health, as one might at first assume, but rather one of the first indications of a disarrayed ego.

Sara enjoyed her work at the bank and was responsible for keeping up the accounts and entering data into the computer. She was obsessed over the details and would spend many extra hours calculating and recalculating to make sure that she did things correctly. She was awkward socially. Most coworkers did not like her. They left her alone and thought of her as "odd." She preferred this and did not accept invitations to lunch or parties when she occasionally got them. Her supervisor respected her ability to get work done.

Sara had been employed for a full year when things fell apart. It started one day when she was entering numbers into the computer. Suddenly, a voice from nowhere said to her "Sara, you no-good, lazy bitch. I know you're embezzling these funds." She believed that her computer was talking to her even though she knew it was not equipped with that function. She was frightened. Someone or something thought she was embezzling funds.

That night Sara could not sleep. All she thought of was the accusatory voice. The next day, she felt worse. She became convinced that the FBI had implanted a device into her computer to monitor her. The device was able to detect every action she made. Sara also thought that she heard her coworkers whispering about her. In her apartment, she heard voices discussing her plan to embezzle funds from the bank. She was afraid to undress or go to the bathroom because she believed FBI cameras had been set up in her apartment. She stopped taking showers and changing her clothes so that the

FBI would not see her naked. Usually immaculately groomed, Sara began to look disheveled.

She was afraid to touch her computer at work. Her mother suspected something was wrong when Sara did not answer her phone. When she went to Sara's apartment and found her huddled in a corner with her hands over her ears, she took Sara to the ER. Psychiatrists hospitalized Sara for three weeks. They determined that Sara was having her first psychotic break. She was put on 10 mg Zyprexa and sent back to work. She did well and did not have another breakdown for two years until she tried to stop her medicine.

DISCUSSION

Sara illustrates many of the aspects of a person with schizophrenia. Premorbidly, she did have a personality disorder—Obsessive-Compulsive Personality Disorder. She was perfectionistic, orderly, and rigid with excessive work patterns, preoccupied with details. She was also introverted and withdrawn. Her lack of ego functioning allowed her to be satisfied with people finding her indistinguishable. She was a good worker and admired by her supervisor. Individuals with schizophrenia often do exceptionally well on tasks that do not require social interaction, like computer programming.

Like Sara, most individuals with schizophrenia have an onset during adolescence or early adulthood. Sara's illness was present for six months after which she had the usual psychotic symptoms. The voice telling her that she was embezzling funds was an auditory hallucination. Her delusions included the idea that the FBI was monitoring her. Sara's behavior was inappropriate as she tried to hide her psychosis. She laughed as she heard the voices and she would grimace in response to them. Her office work suffered because she was afraid to touch the computer. Coworkers talked about her to some extent, since she behaved so strangely. Sara withdrew further. She had positive symptoms of hallucinations, delusions, and strange behavior as well as negative symptoms of restricted emotion, alogia, and avolition.

Schizophrenia has a worldwide prevalence of about 1%. It is known that schizophrenics have a decreased functioning in work, interpersonal relations, and self-care. Since the 1960s, we have had effective medications for treatment. Medications work to decrease dopamine which is thought to cause psychosis. With the newer atypical antipsychotics we are able to get patients back to work and sometimes into relationships and improve their self-care.

Sara's Obsessive-Compulsive Personality Disorder faded when her psychosis was in full bloom, but when she returned to her previous functioning, it returned. In a way, the Obsessive-Compulsive Personality Disorder held her together and allowed her to function at a better level.

Personality Disorders and Obsessive-Compulsive Disorder

Essential Points
- Do not confuse Obsessive-Compulsive Disorder (OCD) with Obsessive-Compulsive Personality Disorder (OCPD).
- Any personality disorder can also have OCD, although histrionic personality disorder would be the least likely.
- OCD is basically an anxiety disorder.
- A patient may have both OCD and OCPD.

OCD patients often perceive their symptoms as invaders from outer space. These unwanted invaders change the course of their lives.
—Drs. Eugen Neziroglu and Jose A. Yaryure Tobias

To have Obsessive-Compulsive Disorder (OCD), your patient needs to have obsessions or compulsions that are severe enough to take up more than 1 hour a day or cause marked distress. Obsessions are persistent ideas, thoughts, or impulses that are intrusive or inappropriate. They are not egosyntonic. Your patient has to think these thoughts and recognize them as from his or her own mind. If the patient feels they are imposed from someone or something, as in thought insertion, it is not OCD. Patients often ruminate about cleanliness and order and they try to suppress these thoughts. Compulsions are repetitive behaviors to reduce anxiety, like hand washing or counting. Compulsions are not connected in any realistic way to the event your patient is trying to prevent.

Obsessive-Compulsive Personality Disorder (OCPD) is not characterized by the presence of obsessions or compulsions and instead involves a preoccupation with orderliness, perfectionism, and control, and begins by early adulthood.

Patients can have eating disorders, trichotillomania (hair-pulling), obsessions about drugs, be hypochondriacs, have paraphilias, or guilty ruminations in the presence of Major Depressive Disorder and still be classified as having OCD if they are not just obsessed with their eating, hair-pulling, and so on.

A Paranoid Personality Disorder will obsess about people being not loyal or untrustworthy if OCD is present on Axis I. A patient with Schizoid Personality Disorder can be compelled to always choose solitary activities. The Schizotypal Personality Disorder can obsess that people are always negative when referring to him, whereas the Antisocial Personality Disorder can compulsively act as if everyone is always positive toward him even when he is conning others. Borderline Personality Disorders can compulsively act out anger toward others.

The Histrionic Personality Disorder tends to be more impulsive than compulsive, but sometimes she can compulsively speak in a certain way to draw attention to herself. They are the least likely to have OCD on Axis I.

Narcissistic Personality Disorder patients may obsess in fantasies of their great beauty or intelligence. Avoidant Personality Disorders can compulsively avoid other people. Dependent personalities can obsessively wait for others to help them.

For the patients who have OCD and OCPD, their preoccupations with order can turn into obsessions and compulsions. OCPD patients can be such perfectionists that they are compelled to keep trying to complete a project, but never achieve it like Sisyphus rolling the proverbial stone uphill.

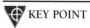 KEY POINT

If your patient is rigid or stubborn, but not obsessing or compelled, only diagnose OCPD.

Remember to rule out behaviors that reflect habits or customs that are culturally sanctioned by the patient's group. For example, if your patient's religious group requires him to wash his hands three times before he eats, do not think that he has OCD unless he is washing 12 times a day and his family and friends are complaining about him.

CLINICAL VIGNETTE

At first sight anyone would think that Mark had the perfect life. He was a tall, handsome, immaculately groomed, 35-year-old attorney with his own practice employing two secretaries and a clerk.

Mark, however, struggled with OCD. One obvious symptom was his need to check and recheck his work obsessively. His excruciatingly slow work speed resulted in his taking three times as long as most attorneys to do a job. Although he would start working at 6 a.m., he often would not finish until after 10 p.m. even if his caseload was light.

His employees thought that Mark was strange. They watched him and often were asked to help him perform certain rituals each day. Before sitting down at his desk, Mark felt compelled to arrange his pens and books in a circular pattern. He could not begin work if the pattern was not set. He required his employees to place files on his desk in sets of two and to only enter his office from the right side of the room. They did not know that Mark was concerned with the symmetrical wear of his rug. Six months earlier he had asked them to only enter from the left side.

Once when a secretary moved a book off his desk, Mark had a fit of rage: he could not work until the book was back on his desk. His staff did not know that he was often irritable and had mood swings and chronic feelings of emptiness. His relationships were intense and unstable to the point where he could also be classified as having Borderline Personality Disorder.

Mark's employees were usually careful to obey his bizarre requests and they spent a lot of time keeping things in the order he liked.

Mark had difficulty leaving his office each night even if his work was done. He always felt as if he had left some essential task uncompleted. One day Mark could not stop checking a bill he had reviewed repeatedly. He would realize that the bill added up correctly and then he would immediately doubt the result. He wasted 3 hours and forgot that an important application was due that day. The incident propelled him into treatment.

Mark visited a psychiatrist who diagnosed OCD and BPD. Mark was prescribed Lexapro, which he had to increase to 60 mg and take for 6 weeks before he felt some relief. He stopped his checking rituals and his time spent working on each case was reduced by 50%.

DISCUSSION

OCD is relatively common, affecting six million Americans. The disorder occurs equally in males and females and often runs in families.

Some researchers have determined that the brain's cingulum is overreactive in OCD. Many patients respond well to antidepressants, especially SSRIs. This supports the theory that OCD is due to a problem with the neurotransmitter serotonin in particular. Behavioral and cognitive therapies can also be useful in treating OCD patients. Behavioral therapy is more useful in dealing with compulsions than in changing obsessive thoughts.

Mark's case is typical of patients with OCD. He was a successful attorney working too many hours involved in compulsive, repetitive behaviors to satisfy his unrelenting obsessions. Even though he was in the office many hours, his OCD prevented him from accomplishing much. The positive aspect of his disorder was tenacity. Once he started a project he never quit until it was done. Medication did not eliminate his persistence—it only made him more efficient. After several months of treatment, Mark's obsessive-compulsive symptoms were reduced by 75%. His anger and mood swings also decreased but not enough to eliminate his Axis II, BPD diagnosis.

Personality Disorders and ADHD

A temperamental constellation consisting of high activity level and short attention span should be first considered.

—Kaplan and Sadock's
Synopsis of Psychiatry, on ADHD

Attention-Deficit/Hyperactivity Disorder (ADHD) is a pattern of inattention and/or hyperactivity and impulsivity present before the age of 7. Many times, the diagnosis is not made until your patient is 10, 11, or even in his or her teen years. Some patients are diagnosed in their adult years. Personality disorders are mostly diagnosed when your patient is an adult. Impairment must be present in ADHD, either in the home or at school or at work. Inattention at school usually leads to poor grades. At work, failure to pay attention leads to messy productions and disorganization. If sustained efforts are needed, then your ADHD patient will have trouble.

Obsessive-Compulsive Personality Disorder (OCPD) would be useful to your ADHD patient, but not many of them have OCPD. Instead, Antisocial Personality Disorder is more common in the ADHD patient. It is easier for an impulsive, inattentive individual to disregard or violate the rights of others and fail to conform to social norms. Irresponsibility and inconsistent work behavior might not be that big a step for your ADHD patient. This is not to say that all ADHD patients will have Antisocial Personality Disorder. Most of them will not lie or con others or physically fight with other people.

Conduct disorder is a pattern of behavior in which the basic rights of others are also violated. There is aggression to people and animals, destruction of property, theft. Patients can have the onset in childhood or adolescence and if they are over 18, they probably have antisocial personality disorder.

In Borderline Personality Disorder patients with ADHD as well, the unstable relationships we usually see are exaggerated. Of course impulsivity is at high levels. Patients with both disorders will spend carelessly, engage in dangerous sex, reckless driving, and binge eating. The risks of suicidal behaviors increase as well. ADHD would be on Axis I, while borderline personality disorder would be classified on Axis II.

In the patient with ADHD and Histrionic Personality Disorder, there is a striving to be the center of attention and provocative behavior. Emotions are rapid and shifting. Intimacy is difficult for histrionic personalities and for ADHD patients. They both have impaired relationships. Delayed gratification is something both groups find challenging. ADHD patients constantly seek novelty, and those with histrionic personality disorder do as well.

KEY POINT

If your patient is self-defeating, think of ADHD and Self-Defeating Personality Disorder.

CLINICAL VIGNETTE

Chuck, a 32-year-old book editor, had a reputation for acquiring brilliant new work and helping coworkers. So strong were his skills that Chuck's boss overlooked his other habits—chronic lateness, a disheveled office, and an inability to follow through—at least for the time being.

At meetings, fellow staff members always expected Chuck to arrive at least 20 minutes past the designated time. New writers and visitors and others were inevitably disappointed if they anticipated punctuality for scheduled appointments. Forgotten assignments were left undone. Careless mistakes marred his mostly excellent work.

When his senior editor entered Chuck's office, which he rarely did, he found Chuck's desk a complete mess, strewn with manuscripts, books, notepads, and pens.

"How can you find anything in here?" his boss asked.

"Don't worry. I know where everything is," Chuck replied.

"Can I have the Patton manuscript?"

Chuck jumped up and nervously rummaged through an unbalanced pile of papers on the edge of his tiny desk.

"Maybe it's on my windowsill."

He ran over and shuffled through another unruly pile. "The author e-mailed most of it too." Chuck sat down at the computer and started clicking away.

"Bring it over when you find it," his boss said as kindly as possible, wondering how he tolerated such a distracted, disorganized worker, regardless of his acquisition record.

Later that afternoon, his boss called Chuck to request the manuscript again. Chuck, in his self-defeating way, had forgotten all about it, even though he knew his boss was looking to cut the number of workers in their department.

The next day Chuck picked up one of his company's latest releases on ADHD. The author was describing Chuck's problems—lack of attention to details, careless mistakes, inability to listen and follow through, disorganized behavior, reluctance to engage in tasks that require sustained mental effort, losing things, and forgetfulness. (The author did not describe Chuck's self-defeating behavior.) At the end of the book Chuck found a list of psychopharmacologists.

When Chuck went to one for an evaluation, he received a diagnosis of ADHD and Self-Defeating Personality Disorder. The doctor gave him Adderall 10 mg XR twice daily. After two weeks, he was able to find manuscripts more easily, clean up his office and apartment, remember important dates, and concentrate on his boss's instructions. Of course, he still defeated himself with constant lateness and saying inappropriate things at meetings.

Chuck had a late adult diagnosis of ADHD, as often happens with bright individuals who use other talents to overcome their deficits. The prevalence of ADHD is about 3% to 7% in school-aged children. The prevalence in adulthood is not currently known, but the diagnosis is becoming more common. Males have ADHD more frequently than females: in a ratio of 4:1 or higher. It is more common in first-degree biological relatives. Genetic studies are needed to determine whether this is due to genes or environment. Study of the neurobiology of ADHD began in 1971 with the exploration of dopaminergic and noradrenergic pathways. Researchers hypothesized that weak frontocortical inhibitory control over subcortical function might be the mechanism for ADHD. To date, CTs and MRIs have found decreased volume in frontal cortex, cerebellum, and subcortical structures. When stimulants like Adderall are used, they block reuptake of dopamine and norepinephrine at neurons, thereby increasing their availability. There are many challenges to treating a patient like Chuck.

21

Personality Disorders and Dementia

> **Essential Concepts**
> • Dementia may result from many causes, i.e., Alzheimer's, vascular, Parkinson's, Huntington's, general medical conditions, Lewy body, etc.
> • Dementias may strengthen or weaken the symptoms of a personality disorder.
> • A personality *change* is different from a personality disorder.
> • Delirium and amnesia are different from dementia.

It it likely that as individuals age, there may be an exacerbation of personality dysfunction because of loss, increased stress, economic disadvantage, and the impact of aging and declining health.

> —*Handbook of Personality Disorders*,
> ed. Jeffrey Magnavita

Dementia is characterized by multiple cognitive deficits. There is memory impairment, aphasia, apraxia, agnosia, and a disturbance in executive functioning. Aphasia is an inability to speak, read, and/or write. Apraxia is an inability to move as the patient wants to move, whereas agnosia is an impairment in recognizing objects. Executive functioning involves the ability to plan, initiate, and stop complex behaviors as well as abstract thinking.

KEY POINT

Memory impairment is both an early symptom and a late one.

Your dementia patients won't be able to learn new things and they will forget what they knew. They will lose keys and valuable possessions as well as their ways when they try to get around familiar neighborhoods. Sometimes, their memories are so poor that they will forget who their family members are or their own names.

Of course, all of this cognitive dysfunction will lead to social and occupational problems. Patients won't be able to work, shop, dress, bathe, and do other activities of daily life.

The age of onset of dementia depends on the cause, but it is usually late in life. Prevalence rates are about 1.5% in people aged 65 to 69 and as much as 16% to 25% for those over the age of 85. Usually, dementia implies a progressive, nonreversible course, but this depends on the etiology.

In Alzheimer's dementia, the deficits begin gradually and keep getting worse. The diagnosis is made only when other dementias are ruled out. At the beginning of this dementia, a paranoid personality disordered patient may get much more distrusting and suspicious, but at the end stages when your patient is worse he may lose his paranoia entirely.

A Schizoid Personality Disorder will withdraw further from others. In the last stages of Alzheimer's, he may be completely indifferent to others or in some cases he may allow others to get closer to him. Schizotypals may be more delusional at first and then become completely eccentric as they degenerate. Antisocial personalities can become extremely aggressive and impulsive throughout the course of the dementia. Borderline Personality Disorders are especially difficult because they will fight more and at times become quite paranoid. Often they will strike out at others or try to hurt themselves.

Histrionic personalities will draw attention to themselves by acting out with shifting emotions. The narcissistic personalities will expect others to serve them all the time while they assume a haughty attitude. Avoidant personalities will keep away from others at the beginning of the dementia, but as it progresses they may very well engage with caretakers because feelings of inadequacy will decrease as cognitive function declines. Dependent Personality Disorders will lean heavily on caretakers until they no longer are able to recognize the need to do so. Obsessive-compulsives will obsess even more as they become impaired, but over time they lose the capacity to do so.

Vascular dementia patients were formerly called multi-infarct dementia patients. They are similar to Alzheimer's patients, also suffering from memory impairment and aphasia, apraxia, agnosia, and decrease in executive functioning. In addition, they have focal neurological signs and symptoms, like increased deep tendon reflexes, gait abnormalities, etc., because various parts of their brains are infarcted—i.e., destroyed by lack of blood flow by clogged arteries. Various personality disorders will be affected as described for Alzheimer's patients. In Lewy Body Dementia, dopamine neurons are destroyed and visual hallucinations may be prominent. Interestingly, the personality disorders are affected as they are in the other dementias.

CLINICAL VIGNETTE

For 20 years, Elvira owned her own Italian restaurant. The 62-year-old started as a waitress, worked her way up to manager, and finally bought the business. She was known as a tough business woman who had fights with workers, adored customers, and loved to overeat, drive recklessly, and drink too much. Her restaurant meant everything to her, especially since she had no "significant other" or immediate family. One evening a favorite customer came in for dinner. Elvira seated him graciously as usual, but called him Ted instead of Will. He was deeply offended because Elvira had always remembered his name in the past as well as what he liked to eat. Another time Elvira failed to pay two waitresses their usual salaries. They were upset and complaining. Elvira apologized and asked them to accompany her to her office. There she puttered around looking for the safe combination. The two women exchanged surprised glances. They had never seen Elvira forget the combination. She finally found the paper with the numbers and opened the safe. Elvira counted and recounted the money. If there was one thing Elvira could do, it was count money. The two waitresses asked her what was wrong, but Elvira denied any problem. They had to help Elvira figure out their salaries.

Customers and staff also noticed that Elvira could no longer tell time or name simple objects such as plates and glasses. Everyone thought it was senility. A distant cousin was called in to help. After several months of negotiations, the assistant manager bought her restaurant and Elvira was placed in a nursing home. When the two waitresses went to visit her six months later in the nursing home, Elvira failed to recognize them. She called one "momma" and the other "sissy."

DISCUSSION

This presentation is typical of dementia of the Alzheimer's type (AD). Elvira had early onset since she was under age 65. Alzheimer's is more prevalent in women than in men. Elvira's was uncomplicated, because it was not accompanied by delirium, delusions, or depression. AD is slowly progressive, which means that Elvira probably had her disorder for many years before anyone noticed. People probably noticed her borderline personality disorder much more. Her anger, aggression, and splitting of people into good ones (customers) and bad ones (certain staff) were overwhelmingly evident. She had more acting out at the beginning of her dementia and she became quieter and more withdrawn as it progressed. The cause of AD is unknown. Microscopic changes in the brain include neurofibrillary tangles and senile plaques. Gross anatomic findings are reduced volume in the frontal and temporal lobes. Autopsy is the only way to make a definitive diagnosis of AD. Individuals with Down's syndrome have an increased prevalence of AD and they get AD in their forties.

Personality changes are affective instability, poor impulse control, outbursts of rage, marked apathy, and paranoia. Elvira had all of these, but her borderline personality disorder could account for them as well. The fact is that these were not new symptoms for her. If they were and the onset began in her sixties, we would say that she had a personality change, but she had an Axis II personality disorder. Many patients with the various forms of dementia get personality changes, but the clinician must be sure that they did not have a personality disorder to begin with.

Delirium, a fixed, false belief, is a disturbance of consciousness accompanied by a change in cognition, not usually starting with dementia. If Elvira gets delirious, then it will develop over a short period of time and be something she can go in and out of and probably caused by some additional medical condition (e.g., an overdose of medicine).

Amnesia is memory impairment, usually not in the context of delirium or dementia.

Personality Disorders and Eating Disorders

Essential Concepts
- Any one with a personality disorder can also have an eating disorder.
- Eating disorders include Anorexia Nervosa and Bulimia Nervosa.
- Borderline, Histrionic, Obsessive-Compulsive, and Narcissistic Personality Disorders are the most likely to have an eating disorder too.
- Many patients with eating disorders also suffer from major depression.

> I ate the whole pie, then a box of cookies, then two chocolate bars. Of course I threw up.
>
> —A patient with bulimia

Anorexia Nervosa was reported as early as in the 1600s. In current society, it is prevalent and popular. Young girls compete with one another to see who can be the thinnest. Web sites targeted to anorexic patients even give tips on how to outsmart doctors and parents to continue losing weight. Most cases (0.5% to 1% of the affected population) begin in early adolescence. Even young men are increasingly presenting with the disorder. Freud believed that some girls lose their appetite at puberty because of a neurotic fear of sexual activity. Hilda Bruch later described the disorder as a way for a young girl to gain self-control and defeat feelings of ineffectiveness.

Anorexics refuse to maintain a normal body weight. They fear gaining any weight and have misperceptions about the shape of their bodies. Women become amenorrheic, i.e., they lose their periods. Anorexics eat a restricted diet. They see themselves as fat, while the world sees them as skinny. Rarely do anorexic patients go to doctors by themselves. Their families usually force them to go.

Patients with Paranoid Personality Disorder, who are also anorexics, believe people are deceiving them about their body weights and other topics. They bear grudges and believe they are being attacked. If the anorexic is schizoid she will stay away from close relationships and take pleasure in few activities. If she is schizotypal, she can have odd beliefs about why she cannot eat and be eccentric in her behavior. If the anorexic patient has an Antisocial Personality Disorder, then she can shoplift (clothes especially) and be irresponsible with others as well as herself. She won't have any remorse. Borderline Personality Disorder is very common with anorexics. In this case, your patient will frantically avoid any abandonment she can detect. Her relationships will be stormy. Her self-image, especially of her body, will be disturbed. Her impulsivity could extend to substance abuse, reckless driving, and suicide attempts. Histrionic Personality Disorder is also common in anorexics. Your patient will be the center of attention and be inappropriately sexual. Self-dramatization and suggestibility will be high. The Narcissistic Personality Disorder will be grandiose, fantasizing about unlimited beauty if only she is skinny enough. She will be so entitled and exploitative that you will wonder how anyone can bear to be with her. The avoidant personalities will hide somewhere, fearing rejection. Dependent personalities will be under someone else's jurisdiction, like a parent or a husband. She will claim that her parent or husband will abandon her if she does not remain thin. She will be so helpless.

Obsessive-Compulsive Personality Disorder (OCPD) is probably the most probable personality disorder with Anorexia Nervosa. How simple it will be for her to be preoccupied with the perfect weight and constantly be dieting. She will be dedicated to work and productivity. The conscientiousness and inflexibility of the OCPD will perfectly fit in with anorexia.

Your patients with Bulimia Nervosa will binge eat and then vomit or give themselves laxatives to have diarrhea. They are also obsessed with their shape and weight. A *binge* is eating in a discrete period of time an amount of food that is larger than most people could eat. Bulimics consume sweet snacks like ice cream or cake. Most bulimics are ashamed of their disorder and hide it. Paranoid personalities do well with covering up their binges and purges. Schizoids sneak off into corners to eat and get rid of the food. Schizotypals have strange beliefs about their eating activities, e.g., a devil made them get rid of the food. Antisocial Personality Disorder may steal food and then enjoy purging it. Borderline personalities will fight with someone and then throw up in protest. Their intense anger and other emotions are somewhat sedated when they binge. Histrionics will make a big show of not eating in front of all the people for whom they are showing off. Narcissists will exploit others as they center on themselves. OCPDs will measure everything they are eating but then counteract everything by vomiting or defecating.

⊕ KEY POINT

Your bulimic patient may purge with vomiting or diarrhea. If she/he does not purge, they will fast or use exercise to deal with the excessive food load.

CLINICAL VIGNETTE

Anna was pleasant and cooperative at her first interview. She was pale and dressed in so many layers that it was difficult to see how painfully thin she was. Anna was 37 years old. In response to questions about her appetite and two previous hospitalizations, she replied she was o.k. and that there was no need to worry. Her speech was soft, coherent, and correct. She had no history of hallucinations or delusions. It was clear to me that she had Anorexia Nervosa (restricting type) and OCPD. I prescribed Prozac 20 mg per day for two weeks and then we would double it to 40 mg. She questioned me carefully about whether the medicine would cause her to gain weight. I assured her that this antidepressant was one of the few not associated with weight gain. I hoped that the Prozac would reduce her obsessive weighing of herself, her perfectionism, and compulsive restriction of food. After four weeks, she did not gain weight, but she felt better with a more positive outlook and fewer obsessions. After five weeks, she felt safe enough to remove some of her sweaters. (It was summer.) I was not surprised to see her arms were like two broomsticks, but I was concerned. It was difficult to determine whether her weight was low enough to warrant another hospitalization. When at first I tried to find out what she ate for breakfast, lunch, or dinner, she lied to me. Sometimes, a few diet colas and a carrot were the only nourishment she allowed to pass through her lips.

The more I focused on her eating disorder, the more sessions she missed. I concentrated on her interactions at work which was less threatening to her. On the positive side, she did not have bulimia or use laxatives. She avoided recreational drugs and alcohol, even though she was isolated from most other people and had never had a boyfriend for more than 3 months. Anna saw her divorced parents separately a few times per year. Sometimes, she would call her married sister on the phone. She had not had a period for several years. At 13 she had been chubby and the kids at school mocked her. Her controlling, angry mother bought her diet books and they dieted together. Her mother stopped when she reached her desired goal, but Anna kept going, taking the diet to extremes, which made her feel powerful over herself. Her mother had ignored her anorexia until Anna fainted and was taken to the hospital, where the doctors insisted that she be admitted. At 17 she was 5'6" and only 90 lbs! Anna hated to be on the ward because the nurses weighed her daily and if she did not want to eat a certain amount of food or gain a certain amount of weight, she was not allowed to get out of bed. She had her own obsessive routines that they did not let her fulfill. Another patient told her to cheat by drinking five glasses of water before being weighed. Anna put rocks in her bathrobe pockets to tip the scales in her favor too. After discharge, she would not see the psychiatrist for follow-ups. She had gone up to 108 pounds and she could not stand it. When she was 30, she finally went to a psychiatrist voluntarily because she could not sleep. Her weight had dropped back down to 90 lbs. The psychiatrist put Anna on Paxil 20 mg. After four weeks she slept well and felt better, with fewer obsessions, but to her horror she weighed 125 lbs, almost normal for her height. Friends complimented her and a man asked her for a date. Nonetheless, Anna stopped taking her meds because she could not tolerate the weight gain and looking in the mirror to see her fat belly and what she thought were huge thighs.

DISCUSSION

By the time I saw her, seven years later, she met all the criteria for Anorexia Nervosa and OCPD. Establishing rapport and positive transference were essential at the beginning of treatment. Anna constantly threatened to stop treatment. In addition, to pharmacotherapy, a cognitive-behavioral approach with positive reenforcement of eating and weight gain was the best option. We worked with her OCPD to lock in obsessive checking of weight gain instead of loss.

TREATMENT ISSUES

Cluster A Clues

> **Essential Concepts**
> - The personality disorders have been clustered into A, B, and C to make them more understandable.
> - Cluster A consists of Paranoid, Schizoid, and Schizotypal Personality Disorders.
> - People with Cluster A symptoms are considered odd and eccentric.
> - Sometimes people fall into a few clusters and all of them should be listed.

He was the oddest man, but clearly not crazy.
                            —Therapist, on a schizoid patient

Many of the symptoms involved in Cluster A patients, especially schizotypal personality disorders, seem to be inherited. More schizotypal patients are biological relatives of schizophrenic patients. Less schizophrenic relatives are found for those with paranoid or schizoid personality disorders.

If patients are suspicious of everyone, turned inward, or imagining strange things, cluster A symptoms, many ordinary people will shun them and consider them weird. These personality disordered individuals are categorized into one group because they are *almost* like psychotic patients, but the Paranoid, Schizoid, and Schizotypal Personality Disorders usually do not hallucinate (either auditory or visual). They may be delusional, however, either in paranoid beliefs or in magical ones. The paranoid delusions would be entertained by Paranoid Personality Disorders and the magical ones by Schizotypal Personality Disorders.

Schizoid Personality Disorders have restricted the expression of emotions and they withdraw from people, but rarely would they ever be delusional. Patients with Schizoid Personality Disorder do not have schizophrenic relatives. Schizoid patients can have successful work histories. They usually are not engaged with others but are more engaged in self-reverie. They recognize reality without a problem.

Patients with Schizotypal Personality Disorder have cognitive-perceptual disturbances that are similar to those with schizophrenia. There is a reduced perfusion or prefrontal brain areas in both Schizotypal Personality Disorder and schizophrenia. Schizotypal Personality Disorder patients have larger lateral ventricle areas like schizophrenics.

Cluster A patients are associated with more suicide risks and homicide attempts. If patients are withdrawn, paranoid, and delusional, there is more of a chance that they will hurt themselves or others. If the patient is older, unmarried, and male, then his risk is further increased. A past suicide attempt is the best indicator that a patient is at risk for suicide. Many suicides are preventable and we must be alert to signs of suicidal ideation in our patients.

 KEY POINT

Always ask if your patient is thinking about hurting himself or anyone else.

Paranoid Personality Disorder patients can be aggressive toward others in their mistaken beliefs that others are "out to get them." Their constant anger, hostility, and resentment can turn into homicide. Schizoid patients are not that involved with others, so they tend to have a lower rate of involvement with homicide. Schizotypal Personality Disorder patients can become paranoid and aggressive. Some of their odd or magical thinking may lead them to act aggressively toward others.

Usually, people act out against family members or people known to them. More than 50% of those who commit homicide have used alcohol beforehand. Cluster A patients can use excessive alcohol or other drugs, although they are not necessarily known for alcoholism or excessive use of alcohol.

CLINICAL VIGNETTE

Andrew was no ordinary 24-year-old. His talents were many. Besides being a superb dancer, he was able to play the piano, sing, and perform magic tricks. However, he never gave himself any credit and no matter how many people complimented him it never registered. He thought of himself as inadequate and inferior to his peers. Since he was taciturn and withholding, no one knew about Andrew's low self-esteem. He would simply put on a performer's smile. He had been raised by a strict maternal grandmother who encouraged him to maintain the family's blue-blood integrity by "keeping a stiff upper lip." Andrew never revealed to anyone that he was born to a heroin-addicted mother who had only had a brief relationship with his father, a famous musician. Instead, he invented a story about a staid, middle-class family. For a short period, Andrew was a member of a modern dance troupe, where many people—men and women—tried to have relationships with him. It was never clear what his sexual preferences were, however, after much agonizing, he refused everyone. Later his solitary nature and refusal to cater to internal politics eventually drove him out of the dance troupe all together.

One Christmas, Andrew became aware of an emptiness inside, which grew to such an overwhelming degree that he could not eat or sleep normally. His mood was so depressed; hence, he went to a local clinic. A third-year psychiatry resident there prescribed an antidepressant that he could not tolerate, because it made him nauseous and hyperactive. He stopped it quickly and never went back to the clinic.

Andrew resigned to commit suicide. He considered this plan the only alternative to his constant suffering. He said nothing to his grandmother whom he called every week. One evening he simply went home and drank cyanide. Everyone who knew him was totally shocked at his death.

DISCUSSION

What caused Andrew to commit suicide and how could his death have been prevented? Mood disorders are the diagnoses most often associated with suicide. Depressed patients commit suicide early in the course of the illness. They tend to be male, single, socially isolated, and older than 45 years. Having a cluster A personality disorder increases the risk of suicide by leading to an absence of or difficulty in relationships. Cluster A's also have trouble adapting to adverse circumstances.

Andrew had the classic symptoms of major depression: disturbed sleep, difficulty eating, depressed mood, low self-esteem. However, his depression was complicated by his Cluster A personality disorder, a Schizoid Personality Disorder. He did not want close relationships, including sexual ones. He was mostly solitary. He lacked close friends to confide in. Even his grandmother did not really have his confidence. He was cold and detached. If Andrew had just been depressed, he might have been able to bond with the third-year resident in the clinic and accept another antidepressant, instead of avoiding her. A more experienced clinician might have been able to engage him or have questioned Andrew about suicidal ideation.

It is particularly egregious that Andrew had contact with a mental health provider and yet was neither helped nor saved from suicide. This is not uncommon: studies have shown that about 20% of people who die from suicide have had contact with mental health providers within a month of their deaths.

The resident mistakenly thought Andrew was at low risk because of his young age, good health, and lack of previous suicide attempts. Also he did not have alcohol or drug dependence. Studies now show that suicide risk among 15- to 24-year-olds has increased considerably.

Cluster B Clues

24

Essential Points
- Cluster B consists of Antisocial Personality Disorder, Borderline Personality Disorder, Narcissistic Personality Disorder, and Histrionic Personality Disorder.
- Individuals with these disorders are considered dramatic, emotional, and erratic.
- Patients can span a few different clusters.
- Transference and countertransference issues are powerful for Cluster B patients.

I never met a borderline patient I did like.

—Psychiatry professor

Antisocial Personality Disorder begins with conduct disorder in childhood and does not improve as patients mature as many other conditions do. Most children with conduct problems do not develop Antisocial Personality Disorder, but for those who do, they cannot respect the law, they are deceitful, impulsive, and aggressive. Their lack of remorse makes them unique. They have Antisocial Personality Disorder. Current research is showing prefrontal abnormalities in MRI studies. Antisocial Personality Disorder patients have lower prefrontal gray matter volumes and dysfunction in their amygdalas. Nevertheless, over time it is believed that these patients may have less impulsive behavior, less arrests, and less fraudulent activities.

KEY POINT

Borderline personality disorder patients first present in early adulthood, although researchers are attempting to trace their behaviors back to childhood.

Children who are diagnosed with Borderline Personality Disorders do not necessarily grow up to be adults with the disorder. Many psychiatrists realize that Borderline Personality Disorder and Antisocial Personality Disorder are not as different as they seem. Both of them have impulsive aggression and family dysfunction. Borderline patients tend to see themselves as victims of aggression while antisocial personalities view themselves as perpetrators of aggression.

Narcissistic Personality Disorder and Histrionic Personality Disorders do not have as much data collected on them. Narcissists tend to manipulate but not with criminal intent. Histrionics are similar to borderline personalities but they are much less impulsive and have less emotional instability.

Most patients with antisocial personalities do not do well at work or socially. Borderline personality patients do better; histrionics and narcissists probably do even better, but all of them are known for their dramatic and erratic presentations. There is room for improvement in the Cluster B patients, unlike the Cluster A or C patients.

CLINICAL VIGNETTE

Before even one appointment with the psychiatrist, the patient, a 27-year-old psychology graduate student, called several times to change the day or time of her first meeting. The doctor did not have any other days available that week, but offered a few slots the following month. No, she said, it was urgent, and she would keep Monday, but could they meet at a different time? Again the doctor could not accommodate her and suggested the next month. They finally kept the appointment on the date and at the time originally scheduled.

She arrived 15 minutes early and impatiently paced the waiting room. Even though she was a student of psychology, the patient did not seem to understand that showing up early could be as significant as coming late for an appointment. By the time she was seated across from the psychiatrist she was furious. As she spoke, she cried profusely, telling a story of chronic depression starting in adolescence and growing acute during her undergraduate years. When the psychiatrist offered tissues, the patient grabbed the box out of the doctor's hand. "It's about time you did something right," she complained.

"What do you feel I've done wrong?" he asked.

"You couldn't give me the appointment I wanted and you seem so uncaring." She pulled her shoulder-length, straight, black hair into a ponytail with a clip, sat up straight, and blew her nose loudly.

She was the daughter of a famous cardiologist and expected to be treated like royalty by most doctors. Her father was a difficult and demanding man who almost divorced her mother, a passive, excessively sweet woman, several times. The patient and her younger brother had suffered through emotional (but not physical) abuse from her father. Because of him, she concluded, she developed horrible feelings of inadequacy, even though she was a straight-A student, a superb tennis player, and an accomplished pianist.

She was in her second episode of depression, but did not want to take antidepressants again (she had been on Paxil) because she was finally in her longest-yet relationship with a man (6 months) and she wanted to avoid sexual dysfunction. Her sleep was poor and interrupted by panic attacks in the early morning. She had lost 15 pounds and felt irritable, anxious, and melancholic every day. The psychiatrist wanted her to try Lexapro 10 mg and wrote her the prescription. At the end of the session, the psychiatrist asked her for payment as they had agreed when they originally scheduled the appointment. She said her father should be sent the bill. The doctor reminded her of their agreement for the future and said this time he would bill her father, but he wanted her to pay after each appointment.

Before the next visit, a week later, she called several times once again. The psychiatrist tried to reassure her about all the problems for which she complained. Her father called finally and asked the psychiatrist to reduce the bill because his daughter was so "special." The psychiatrist said no. The patient never called to reschedule, but never showed up for the second appointment.

DISCUSSION

This patient has two of the cluster B personality disorders: borderline and narcissistic. She also has major depression and panic disorder, which are easier to treat. In this case, the patient engaged the doctor from the beginning in a frantic, demanding way. In a grandiose way, she wanted to be seen on her schedule. Even though she had never met the doctor she was afraid of abandonment. If she could force him to see her earlier, that would demonstrate that he was available to her and that she was "special." With other people clearly this would be a way of setting up unstable, intense relationships, because no one could fulfill these unvoiced, unreasonable needs. The doctor was immediately devalued in her mind and seen as uncaring when he did not obey her wishes. In the future, he could easily be seen as wonderful and idealized, if he complied. The patient was angry with him even though she was the one who came early and made herself wait. She had affective instability and thought of herself as inadequate many times. Narcissists can feel this way at times, especially if they also have Borderline Personality Disorder as well.

The doctor realized what kind of patient he was dealing with very quickly. He knew he had to set firm boundaries of time, place, and fees. He tried to keep the original appointment and the original conditions of payment at the time of the visit. The patient, not surprisingly, tried to break these boundaries. When she could not break them herself, she engaged her father who unknowingly fell into the struggle.

The patient did not set out to consciously break boundaries or give her doctor a difficult time. Her behavior was unconsciously motivated. If asked, she would have said the world was hostile and abandoning and she was entitled to respect. She may also have been exhibiting projective identification, a defense in which the Borderline Personality Disorder patient projects unwanted aspects of herself on to another person and then acts out with that person.

The psychiatrist may get frustrated and angry with this acting-out Cluster B patient. He should remember to constantly monitor his countertransference feelings, which can be intense and negative. Many times, therapists must have supervision or their own therapy to be able to deal with Cluster B patients.

Cluster C Clues

> **Essential Points**
> - Cluster C consists of the Avoidant, Dependent, and Obsessive-Compulsive Personality Disorders.
> - Individuals with these disorders are considered anxious or fearful.
> - Clustering has considerable limitations and has not been seriously validated.
> - Medical conditions that can cause Cluster C must be ruled out.

> I will throw myself into the grave with her when she dies.
>
> —A patient with Dependent Personality Disorder when asked what she would do when her mother died

People with Cluster C Personality Disorders have excessive fearfulness, inhibition, and anxiety about social interactions. Classical studies have been carried out with pre-Kindergarten children playing in a room with a one-way mirror. Researchers observe the children who are unaware of being observed. Even at this early stage, the potentially Cluster C children will be isolated and on the periphery of the room, afraid to play with others. More normal children will be in the center of the room interacting with others. These inhibited traits appear early in development and are stable over time. An anxious temperament can lead to Avoidant or Dependent Personality Disorder. Cluster C people can cling to family members or lack confidence in their activities. Obsessive-Compulsive

Personality Disorder patients were probably hardworking, unemotional, and perfectionists as children. However, the research has not been carried out to see if this is true.

Avoidant Personality Disorder patients have a terrible fear of being criticized or rejected in social situations. They tend to be shy, quiet, and inhibited. They are afraid to react to others, whereas Dependent Personality Disorder patients go to excessive lengths to get others to care for them. Dependent Personality Disorder people are anxious and fearful too, but they solve their anxiety by leaning on others. Obsessive-compulsive disorder patients are mostly preoccupied with interpersonal control and being orderly and perfect. They do not easily work with others or submit to others because of their fears of losing control.

The brain structure most frequently implicated in fear and anxiety is the amygdala. This area responds to fearful stimuli and connects to emotionally linked memories.

Cluster C patients want to "avoid harm" at all costs. Whether they view other people as causing harm or have fear of new situations or new tasks, they have the personality dimension of harm avoidance. These patients tend to remain stable over time.

✪ KEY POINT

Clustering of these personality disorders is only one way to categorize them and it limits a full view of the personality disorders.

Validation of clustering has not been performed and many clinicians are skeptical of this viewpoint with good cause. Research needs to be carried out in each field to document the validity of diagnostic entities. This has not been carried out with Cluster C disorders. The most work has been done with regard to Cluster B's, Borderline Personality disorder in particular.

Medical conditions are especially important to rule out in the Cluster C diagnoses. Avoidant personalities may have concurrent use of alcohol or marijuana, which may cause them to withdraw from others. Dependent personalities may have epilepsy, diabetes, metabolic syndromes, or other medical conditions that cause them to rely on others excessively at the beginning of their lives. Many of these patients are never trained to rely on themselves even though it would be possible. Obsessive-compulsive personalities could have a condition like cocaine addiction or Tourette's or other medical conditions causing them to be overly conscientious and inflexible.

CLINICAL VIGNETTE

The patient, a 56-year-old homemaker, had been married for 34 years. She had neither lived alone nor worked outside the home. Depressed on and off for 4 years before receiving treatment she had warned her family that she would kill herself if her husband ever left her.

The husband, a 58-year-old attorney, had supported her and their two sons for their entire marriage. It was not until he was hospitalized for severe depression himself that he decided to divorce his wife. Through psychotherapy, he realized that he resented his position as sole provider for the whole family. As soon as he was discharged, he served her with divorce papers.

The woman was devastated. A week later, her sons found her sequestered at home, not eating, washing, or engaging in her usual activities. All she wanted to do was sleep, and when awake, she cried and bemoaned her fate. When she threatened to commit suicide, her sons called the police, who forced her to go with them to the emergency room. She was admitted to a psychiatric ward for depression.

The patient had tried most antidepressants during previous depressive episodes, but the only one that worked was the MAOI, Nardil.

In the hospital, they gave her Effexor 300 mg and discharged her after 2 weeks.

Her psychotherapy began after the hospitalization. When she arrived for her first appointment, she was neatly dressed in casual clothes and appeared her stated age. She cried so hard through the first meeting that it was hard for her to speak. She urgently requested to remain an outpatient, as her inpatient experience had been so dreadful. Her husband had always advised her on the tiniest details of everyday life, from what kind of pasta to cook to how to invest the few funds she controlled. Every session began with her crying hysterically about losing him because she did not know how to live without him. Since her husband had abdicated his role, she wanted her sons to assume responsibility for her.

The plan was to have the patient take care of herself, but she was resistant. The original attraction to her husband was that he was a dominant, take-charge individual who left no room for her own opinions, and she was a lady who just had to worry about where to lunch. Now on the small income to which she had temporarily been reduced, she wondered how she would survive without her luxuries, manicures, designer dresses, and her hair dresser. Her sons assured her that after the divorce finalized, she would still have a considerable fortune and would never need to work.

Her worst times were in the morning when she was alone and feeling dreadful. She could not conceive of how she would be able to take care for herself. A course of study in computer science was suggested because she was barely able to operate her cell phone. In college, she had earned straight A's and graduated with honors with a bachelor's degree in business. Her IQ was higher than average but she had never tried to improve herself. She had relied on her husband, sons, and friends for everything. She only agreed to take a computer course when a friend said she would go with her.

Therapy consisted of structuring the patient's time and teaching her basic skills of living. She was to wake up at a set hour each weekday, make breakfast, attend class, go to the gym, and then have lunch or dinner with one friend or another. It was an enviable life that did not necessitate working, but she could not understand how lucky she was. She remained reluctant to do anything on her own, because she lacked confidence in her abilities. She wanted to jump into another relationship before she dealt with the loss of her husband. She wanted someone else to immediately support and infantilize her. The struggle was to make her aware of her excessive dependency needs.

DISCUSSION

In therapy, the patient attempted to place her psychiatrist in the role her husband had just vacated, expecting him to make all her important decisions and tell her what to do. The doctor resisted this role and instead helped her to initiate projects on her own. Her self-confidence needed to be built-up and she needed the experience of assuming responsibility for herself. The patient's father had died when she was 10 years old. It was a terrible loss as she was so close to him. Her grandmother took over and dominated her and her mother. Both she and her mother were treated like babies who could not do anything on their own.

It was clear that this patient had Dependent Personality Disorder and major depression. She was afraid to get angry with others for fear of alienating them and having them abandon her the way her father had when he died prematurely. When her husband left, it seemed a tragedy and it was hard for her to open up to new ways of thinking and behaving.

26 ▼ Gender Benders

Essential Points
- Certain personality disorders are diagnosed more frequently in men; i.e., Antisocial Personality Disorder.
- Other personality disorders are diagnosed more frequently in women; i.e., Borderline, Histrionic, and Dependent Personality Disorders.
- Differences in prevalence may be real or social stereotypes.
- Notice that women generally are considered more emotional, anxious, and dramatic (Cluster B), so we have Borderline, Histrionic, and Dependent Personality Disorders that are more prevalent in women.
- Men may be allowed to break society's rules and so they may be more antisocial.

Boys don't cry.
> —Main character (who seems to have had
> Borderline Personality Disorder) in the
> 1999 movie of the same name, in which
> a woman was passing for a man.

Men and boys are the ones most frequently diagnosed with Antisocial Personality Disorder. The rates are about 3% in males and only 1% in females. Higher prevalence rates are found in prisons or drug treatment centers. Basically, there is a disregard for and violation of the rights of others in this personality disorder. Boys are socialized differently from girls. Fathers and mothers may disregard aggressive and disrespectful behavior in boys that they would never tolerate in girls. The saying "Boys will be boys" has a lot of meaning in our society. If boys break rules and violate social norms, many parents may think of this as creativity. If girls deviate from the social order, they are usually shamed back into good behavior. Their acting out is not considered creative by most parents. Girls are taught to avoid physical fighting, to be responsible toward others, and to take care of their safety as well as others. All of this social responsibility works against developing sociopathy.

Head injury and abuse are two factors that contribute to antisocial behavior. Boys are usually more active and can have head injury from games and fighting. Abuse can be physical, sexual, or emotional. Most serial killers come from horrible backgrounds where they were abused by their caretakers. Perhaps more boys receive abuse than girls. Researchers have found that physical aggression is inherited. Certain genes that deal with dopamine, serotonin, and various enzymes have been implicated. Perhaps those children, especially boys, with these genes go on to develop Antisocial Personality Disorder. Antisocial children are usually exposed to adverse backgrounds. Aggression, impulsivity, and lack of remorse combine to develop Antisocial Personality Disorder in certain individuals.

⊕ KEY POINT

Women are seen as having more Borderline, Histrionic, and Dependent personalities. Again this could be due to the way we socialize girls and women.

In our society if a girl has a strong emotional reaction to something, it will be reinforced more than if a boy has one. A boy may be called a "sissy" if he cries or complains too loudly about a problem. Impulsivity is an important factor in Borderline Personality Disorder that leads to unstable relationships, a bad self-image, and reckless sex or binge eating. Borderline personalities are always trying to avoid "abandonment." In our culture, it would be "unmanly" for a male to be overly concerned about losing a relationship whereas for women it can be somewhat appropriate. Men usually are less fixated on their self-image. Instead of self-mutilating or suicidal threats, men may actually commit suicide. Trauma and neglect in childhood can lead to borderline pathology in women and antisocial behavior in men. Borderline Personality Disorder is diagnosed about 75% in females and only 25% in males.

Histrionic Personality Disorder includes excessive emotionality and attention seeking behavior. They need to be the center of attention and they can be inappropriately seductive. They use their physical appearance to attract others. Most of these characteristics are associated with women. In clinical settings, this disorder is diagnosed more frequently in females. Some studies, however, report similar prevalence rates in males and females. The male with Histrionic Personality Disorder may "strut his stuff," show off his muscles or his clothes. Because of stereotypes, clinicians tend to classify women in this category more often.

Dependent Personality Disorder is also diagnosed more in women although in some cultures men may also be encouraged to be dependent. These personalities are seen as clinging, submissive, with terrible fears of separation. In our society, if a girl wants to stay at home with her parents, it is not considered unusual. Nevertheless, if a boy wants to do this, he will be discouraged.

 KEY POINT

If a girl is passive and polite, people will think she is pleasant. If a boy has this behavior, his parents will worry about him.

In clinical settings, Dependent Personality Disorder is seen more in women, although research studies are reporting similar prevalence in men and women.

Individuals, both males and females, who have cross-dressed and tried to pose as a male (if a female) or a female (if a male) have been quite surprised by how others treated them. For example, one woman dressed as a boy for a joke and attended a party. She really looked the part, according to friends who were in on the joke. She found herself pushed around physically by "real" men who were not in on the joke and when she tried to make casual body contact with other females, they shrank from her. These physical reactions surprised her. She never realized what she took for granted. Her body language was also telling. She was a modest individual who usually kept her hands folded in her lap and her legs crossed. As a "male" she found she was not comfortable unless she took up more space by spreading her legs when she sat and extending her arms over chairs. Unconsciously, we expect certain behaviors from males and females that are not immediately obvious unless we try to deviate from them. In the movie "Boys Don't Cry," Hilary Swank passes as a boy for a while, but unconsciously other men know something is wrong. When they find out she is a woman, they almost kill her. The way we diagnose personality disorders is influenced by our stereotypes about men and women.

CLINICAL VIGNETTE

Natalie's flair for dressing and her 5'10", 120-pound measurements made her look like a model. Her work as an assistant to a health club manager did not provide her with enough salary to buy real designer clothes, but she shopped at vintage stores and found outfits that glamorized her slender figure and beautiful, long, red hair.

Her personality was irrepressible. One minute she would laugh uncontrollably and the next minute she would cry. Her favorite pastime at the job was flirting with male potential health club members. If her boss wanted to convince a reluctant man to join the club, he would ask Natalie to fawn over him. She was not effective with women who mostly resented her. If any of the men tried to date her, she would reject them immediately. She had been in love twice, but at 25 she was not ready to settle into just any relationship.

One night she and five other employees went out for drinks after work. Natalie sat at the head of the table wearing a well-cut red suit of a perfect shade to match her hair, giggling and sipping her giant martini. She entertained the group with stories, poking fun at her boss and some members. In the ladies' room, Natalie wanted to continue joking with one of her colleagues, but her coworker turned away from her and walked out. Natalie felt rejected. It was not the first time she had misread someone. Often she would think people were her best friends when they were not.

After having too much to drink, Natalie went home by herself to her studio apartment. She changed into a pink satin dressing gown and sat combing her long hair. Suddenly, she heard a voice commanding her to jump out the window. She turned and looked everywhere around her small apartment. There was no one there. The voice then told her to kill herself again. She cried and tried to close off her ears with both hands. Of course, the voice was coming from her own head and she could not stop the sound. She was having auditory hallucinations, triggered by too much alcohol. The next morning she sobered up and felt much better. She did not hear anything further.

DISCUSSION

Natalie had all the classical features of Histrionic Personality Disorder. If she was not the center of attention or flirting with a man, she felt ignored. Her emotions bubbled from one extreme to another. She was theatrical and overexpressive. As indicated by her interaction in the ladies' room, she considered relationships intimate when they were not. Because people with Histrionic Personality Disorder are usually unaware of their true feelings, they exhibit shallow emotional demonstrations, called histrionics. When stressed they can dissociate and lose contact with reality, especially if they drink or use drugs. Natalie had auditory hallucinations as a result of her drinking. These can occur as a result of alcohol or when a vulnerable person is withdrawing from alcohol.

The DSM committees considered changing or eliminating Histrionic Personality Disorder from the DSM-V because they thought it was diagnosed too often in women and that it might be sexual stereotyping. You can imagine a man in Natalie's place but it would probably turn out so differently.

It's Just Culture

Those French people are so cool.
—An American expressing cultural stereotype

It is very difficult to assess personality traits across cultures. To say that Germanic cultures tend to produce more Obsessive-Compulsive Personality Disorders than say Latin cultures would not be accurate. Many psychologists and other scientists have tried to prove that the strict and early toilet training in Northern European cultures, like Germany, Norway, and Finland, induces obsessive traits in their inhabitants. On the other hand, the looser and later toilet training in Southern Europe, i.e., Italy, Spain, France,is supposed to be responsible for Histrionic Personality Disorders. These are vast overstatements, simplifying complex issues.

Three broad personality traits—neuroticism, extraversion, and psychoticism—have been recognized and studied for years. It is believed that neuroticism and extraversion can be measured across cultures, but not psychoticism. In some non-Western cultures, the idea of a personality distinct from others is unknown, so then a personality cannot be studied.

National stereotypes do not always work except to solidify group identity. Statements like, "All Americans love freedom" may be useful for rallying the troops, but inaccurate in describing personalities. When self-esteem is measured, increased extraversion is associated with positive self-esteem and increased neuroticism with low self-esteem in all cultures.

Antisocial Personality Disorder seems to be pervasive in lower socioeconomic groups. This makes sense in an adaptive world view: Why should lower socioeconomic groups respect lawful behaviors and social norms that exclude them? If a 13-year-old boy longs to have a baseball bat and he cannot get one because he has no money, then it makes sense that he steals it. Of course, that will get him arrested or in trouble, but if his parents are unavailable or disrespectful of laws themselves, his behavior is logical.

Paranoid Personality Disorders may be exhibited by minority groups who feel discriminated against in the larger society. If you are the only African-American in your community you might be suspicious, doubting peoples' loyalty, reluctant to confide in others, and you might bear more grudges. This may be true of you if you are a recent immigrant or refugee.

If you move from a town of 300 people to New York City, with 8 million people, you probably will tend to turn inward, not desire close relationships, be indifferent to others, and feel detached. This was known as "emotional freezing." Many immigrants are seen as cold, hostile, indifferent, but they may just be protecting themselves. You could be mistaken for a schizoid personality.

Or what if you were born in Haiti where your family practiced voodoo on a regular basis. Your beliefs could mistakenly get you classified as a Schizotypal Personality Disorder.

Borderline Personality Disorder, on the other hand, seems to be seen around the world. These individuals feel existential dilemmas, anxiety, sexual conflicts, and various social pressures. They react with affective instability, anger, and feelings of emptiness.

Across cultures, human personalities tend to be the same. Cultural differences are vast, but aspects of introversion, extraversion, or psychotism or neuroticism differ.

Personality Disorders and Substance Abuse

Essential Concepts
- Any of the personality disorders can have substance abuse.
- The most common personalities associated with substance abuse are antisocial, borderline, and narcissistic.
- Substance abuse is a maladaptive pattern for 1 year that leads to failure in the home, at work, or in school, in terms of legal and social problems.
- Substance dependence includes tolerance, withdrawal, and compulsive use.
- Substances are alcohol, amphetamines, caffeine, cannabis, cocaine, hallucinogens, opioids, etc.

Well, I woke up this morning, I got myself a beer
Well, I woke up this morning, and I got myself a beer
The future's uncertain, and the end is always near
                        —Jim Morrison, "Roadhouse Blues"

Substances affect mood and behavior and when a patient is "under the influence" he/she can look like he/she has schizophrenia, bipolar disorder, or any psychiatric diagnosis.

Our personality disordered patients do not need any further problems, but they often have them when they abuse various substances. Alcohol and nicotine are the two most commonly abused substances, with marijuana and cocaine not lagging far behind. Men have more substance abuse than women. They also have more diagnoses of Antisocial Personality Disorder. Something like 40% to 50%

of patients with substance abuse or dependence also have Antisocial Personality Disorder. These patients are more impulsive, isolated, and depressed. If a person with Antisocial Personality Disorder is inhibited, then he will fail even further in conforming to social norms, stopping his impulsivity and aggressiveness or being responsible. All of his characteristics, in the first place, will lead him to drink or smoke "crack."

 KEY POINT

Borderline Personality Disorder patients have unstable and intense relationships that upset them. They will often try to modulate their feelings with substances like alcohol or "downers."

Borderline Personality Disorder patients have impulsivity drives them to binge on food or substances. When they feel "empty" and abandoned they might fill up with a drug or drink.

Narcissistic personalities need to maintain their grandiosity, which a substance might improve. They feel they are "special," so of course they cannot get addicted like normal people. They are also entitled to anything they want.

Paranoid Personality Disorders might "need" a drink to relax from their constant vigilance. If they try stimulants or cocaine substances they may find themselves having true paranoia.

Schizoid, avoidant, and dependent personalities may tend to use more opiates. Opiates would turn the schizoid more inward, the avoidant away from others, and cause the dependent to rely on the "pusher" or another substance abuser.

Self-Defeating Personality Disorder patients can constantly sabotage themselves with drugs or alcohol. Schizotypal will become even stranger with marijuana or other substances.

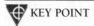 KEY POINT

Personality disordered patients are more difficult to treat for substance abuse.

The first step is to get patients off the drugs. Hospitalization is useful for alcoholics, opiate abusers, and cocaine addicts. Once abstinence has been maintained, then the abusive patterns can be addressed. Often patients need to be in lifelong programs like AA, NA, etc. We know how difficult it is for personality disorder patients to change their patterns. They are stuck and substance abuse may be just one more aspect that cannot be altered.

CLINICAL VIGNETTE

Wanda, a 30-year-old marketing executive, had a secret method of maintaining her exceptionally, slender figure: snorting a few hundred dollars worth of cocaine each day.

She hoped no one would discover her secret, but worried that people would be suspicious of her shakiness and frequent exits during meetings. However, since she felt so "special" and entitled, she was convinced that these telltale signs would be overlooked.

Addicted to cocaine for 6 months, Wanda had started snorting recreationally with her boyfriend on weekends and was proud of never smoking crack. She thought if she only snorted the drug, she could control herself.

Wanda's eventual daily drug use necessitated a constant supply of cocaine, forcing her to drive to a frightening neighborhood to buy drugs.

The pusher, who worked as a stock boy at the bodega where she went, increased his prices. Wanda had to pay whatever he wanted. He would not bargain with her. One night when Wanda came to the bodega he was not there. The owner claimed he never existed. Wanda tried to use her sexual attractiveness to win over the owner, but he was unmoved by her. She felt paranoid with everyone staring at her in the store. She left and never went back. After a long search, she found a man in her office building who sold cocaine, but his prices were double the stock boy's. It did not matter, Wanda paid whatever he asked, including her entire large salary and the mortgage on her condo.

Cocaine did so many things for Wanda, she could not think of living without it. It suppressed her appetite, so she could stay 20 lbs lighter. She could wear the latest fashion and look great. She knew all her girlfriends envied her. She was unbelievable. She could work 12 hours at a stretch and not be tired.

Two or three hours sleep was all she needed. If she felt irritable she just took a hit of coke.

In a meeting with some important clients one day, Wanda felt unfocused and nervous, so she excused herself and ran to the ladies' room for a hit of coke. When she returned she bent eagerly over the papers and blood poured out of her nose. Everyone was solicitous, handing her tissues, and telling her to sit with her head tilted back. The next day, paranoid that people would know what her nosebleed was from, she decided to stop coke.

She was so fatigued and lethargic. In the cafeteria, she chose pancakes and macaroni and cheese, instead of salad and coffee. She gobbled down the starchy food and then ordered chocolate cake. Her head ached. She could not concentrate. She managed to stop the drug for 3 days, but then her pusher gave her a free vial of crack and the use of his pipe. Wanda wanted to resist, but he told her she was getting fat and she needed a hit.

She took his pipe into the ladies' room and got high in minutes. For the next few days, she binged on crack forgetting her principles. She finally went to her primary physician who placed her in a rehab program. Afterward she went to

Narcotics Anonymous, but relapsed six times before she stopped cocaine.

DISCUSSION

Wanda had Narcissistic Personality Disorder, which may have helped to push her into cocaine addiction. She was able to feel grandiose, special, admired, entitled, and arrogant on cocaine.

Cocaine addicts spend a great deal of money on the drugs, so they can easily get involved in theft, drug dealing, and prostitution. The high includes increased vigor, gregariousness, hyperactivity, hypervigilance, and impaired judgment. An ear, nose, and throat specialist found that Wanda had a perforated nasal septum because of snorting.

Wanda's six relapses may seem excessive, but they are not unusual. Her narcissistic personality could work against her recovery. On cocaine she was able to have fantasies of unlimited success and beauty, plus she looked the way she wanted, and was able to be haughty and entitled.

Personality Disorders, PTSD, and Somatoform Disorders

> **Essential Points**
> - A patient with a personality disorder is more likely to experience PTSD.
> - Cluster B patients may manifest PTSD more readily, although Clusters A and C suffer PTSD too.
> - Somatoform disorders are often seen in Avoidant, Paranoid, Self-Defeating, Histrionic, and Obsessive-Compulsive Personality Disorders.
> - Any of the patients with personality disorders may have a somatoform disorder.

Personality disorders are really trauma disorders.
—*Handbook of Personality Disorders*,
ed. Jeffrey Magnavita

Posttraumatic Stress Disorder (PTSD) follows a trauma to which a patient is subjected. The fear is not processed by the person at the time because of the severity of the trauma and/or a result of the patient's mental state. Our patients with personality disorders are not particularly good at processing trauma, so they are more likely to have recurrent, intrusive recollections of the event, dreams about it, and bad reactions to cues about the event. They may become avoidant and have increased arousal about the trauma.

Cluster B patients are more likely to have PTSD. Antisocial personality disorder patients are constantly traumatized because when they break laws and boundaries they get into dangerous situations. Their impulsivity and aggressiveness cause physical fights, as does their disregard of safety precautions. Borderline personalities have intense, unstable relationships that traumatize them. They are impulsive too and wind up in all sorts of trouble. Narcissistic and histrionic personality disorders are excessively emotional and interacting with people in ways that traumatize them.

 KEY POINT

The Cluster A's and C's also have more PTSD than the general population.

Paranoid personalities are naturally hypervigilant and irritable and become more so with PTSD. Schizoid personalities easily detach and restrict themselves while avoidant personalities avoid others and activities very easily. Dependent personalities will cling to their caretakers much more with PTSD. Obsessive-compulsive personalities will concern themselves with controlling and ordering their environments while they are numbed by PTSD.

CLINICAL VIGNETTE

Flying was not something Angie had been afraid of until after the accident. At 33, she was a mother of two with a part-time job as a clerk in a stationery store. One Friday night, Angie and her husband, daughter, and son were flying west on a major airline to visit her mother-in-law for the holidays. It had been a smooth flight until the pilot announced "clear air turbulence." He instructed everyone to fasten their seat belts. Angie heard the announcement in the lavatory and felt the plane bounce a few times. As she made her way back to her seat, the aircraft suddenly dropped hundreds of feet. Before she could orient herself, she hit her head on the ceiling. Angie felt suspended in midair for several seconds, and watched as her children and husband sat safely belted in their seats. A terrible fear and hopelessness overcame her. Events from her life flashed through her mind. Angie soon fell to the floor of the plane, picked herself up, then quickly took her seat, and buckled her seat belt. Her heart pounded violently and she felt extremely anxious. The plane made an emergency landing in the Midwest, where the passengers were all taken to the hospital. The doctor who examined Angie assured her that she was fine except for a banged-up shoulder.

But Angie was not fine. That night she began to experience problems. Usually, a good sleeper, she was unable to fall asleep. Once she did, Angie had a nightmare that her plane crashed and burned her to death. She woke up screaming. Her husband tried to calm her. She pushed him off. The next day her appetite was diminished. She could not stop thinking about how afraid she was of flying. Every time her son dropped a toy or her daughter yelled, she shivered. Her husband teased her about her sensitivity. "I always knew you were high maintenance but this is crazy," he said. At work, her fellow employees were surprised to see her moping around. Finally, her boss suggested that she should consult a doctor. Angie ignored him. She always believed she was "special" and felt entitled to "be" anyway she liked. Two months passed and her sleeping, eating, startle response, mood, and concentration were not normal. Angie reluctantly went to a psychiatrist her friend recommended. The psychiatrist, an empathic woman in her fifties, made Angie feel comfortable. She explained that when people are subjected to distressing events outside the range of common experiences they can develop PTSD. The doctor recommended psychotherapy once a week and daily pharmacotherapy with Zoloft 100 mg per day. During therapy, Angie was able to discuss the horrible fear of dying that she experienced when the plane was falling, which reminded her of several life-threatening accidents she had survived as a child. After 6 months of treatment, Angie felt like herself again. She began to sleep and eat well. She calmed down and concentrated. Of course, she still had a grandiose sense of self-importance, believed she was "special" and needed a lot of admiration. When her husband suggested they fly west to see his mother again, she agreed, whereas 2 months earlier she had vetoed that plan.

DISCUSSION

PTSD is very common. Lifetime prevalence is 1% to 14% of the population. Men are at a higher risk for traumatic exposure than women, yet women more frequently develop PTSD. Usually, patients experience the symptoms within 3 months of the trauma (any life-threatening event). Angie experienced PTSD immediately after the plane accident. She responded with intense fear and hopelessness, two common reactions. Her Narcissistic Personality Disorder probably caused her to be unable to process the trauma in a way in which she could avoid PTSD. Personality disorders stop patients from dealing with trauma correctly, i.e., without blocking feelings and reactions. Her grandiosity made her overestimate her abilities and ruminations led her away from processing her feelings so they were cutoff prematurely and led her to PTSD. Her persistent symptoms of increased arousal, sleep problems, irritability, decreased concentration, and exaggerated startle response were all typical. Fortunately for Angie, she quickly addressed the problem, so she did not develop phobias, major depression, or somatization. Zoloft works well in PTSD as many other SSRIs do. Of course, her Narcissistic Personality Disorder was left intact by her short treatment.

In somatoform disorders, patients have physical symptoms that suggest physical disorders that turn out not to be medical conditions. The symptoms distress our patients and interfere with their lives. Personality disordered people are more likely to have any of the somatoform disorders, which include somatization (called hysteria or Briquet's syndrome) of many physical symptoms, conversion disorder (two neurological complaints), hypochondriasis (worry about disease), body dysmorphic disorder (false belief that a body part is defective), pain disorder (pain as the focus), or undifferentiated (unexplained physical complaints). It is believed that avoidant, paranoid, self-defeating, histrionic, and Obsessive-Compulsive Personality Disorders have the most somatoform disorders. In a way, PTSD is similar to somatoform disorders in that feelings are not processed properly. In PTSD, there is a traumatic event that triggers a suspended state of processing, whereas in the somatoform disorders these traumatic events may have occurred in early childhood or later and the symptoms are mostly settled in the body. The theaters of the body play out the patients' concerns. There is a classical story of a man who wanted to strangle his father who wakes up the next day with a paralyzed hand. This would be called conversion disorder today. Nowadays, when patients are so knowledgeable about psychology we rarely see such dramatic conversions, but in Freud's time they were more common.

CLINICAL VIGNETTE

Barbara, a 38-year-old bakery shop owner, spent more than 3 hours one night worrying about pain in a mole on her cheek. She had had the mole since childhood, but now believed it was cancerous. A visit to the dermatologist, during which the doctor assured her the mole was benign, relieved her fear. The pain soon faded.

One week later, after she had been constipated and then had diarrhea, Barbara was convinced she had bowel cancer. Her primary care physician examined her and determined everything was normal. The doctor did not even think a colonoscopy was necessary. Again Barbara felt better almost immediately. The three employees in Barbara's bakery often smirked behind their boss's back. They joked that Barbara must be "dying of cancer" again. They had been through too many scares about their boss's health to take them all seriously. They were also tired of her being the center of attention all the time and dramatizing everything.

One day, Barbara tasted a chocolate frosting. "Too much sugar," she told the employee who had made it. Soon after Barbara had trouble swallowing and her hands and feet felt numb. "What did you put in there?" she asked the woman. "Remember I told you not to use preservatives." "No," insisted the employee, "no preservatives." Barbara felt terrible for the rest of the afternoon. She was allergic to preservatives and felt her worker had accidentally used them. Barbara went to her doctor again and for the tenth time that year she was told that she was in perfect physical condition. Barbara continued on like this, with one physical complaint after another.

DISCUSSION

Barbara's main symptoms began before she was 30 and had persisted. Her condition was chronic, but fluctuated with different life events. Instead of expressing her real feelings, she would have a physical symptom that could not be fully explained medically. She had a rapid and superficial expression of some emotions because she also had Histrionic Personality Disorder. In order for the diagnosis or somatization disorder (*DSM-IV-TR*) to be made, four of Barbara's symptoms must be linked to the gastrointestinal tract, one must be sexual and one must be pseudoneurologic. She easily fulfilled these criteria. Studies show that the prevalence of somatization disorder is from 0.2% to 2% in women and less than 0.2% in men. It is a disorder that frustrates the patient and the doctor. Patients do not like to visit psychiatrists because they deny that their problems have a psychological component. Many of these patients are anxious and depressed. Doctors need to establish a supportive, caring relationship with the patient. Regularly scheduled appointments that are structured and brief can be helpful. The patient's symptoms should be acknowledged as real, but the physician should stress that there is no particular cure. As in Barbara's case, symptoms can clear quickly after a doctor's visit. Barbara had been sexually molested as a child as many patients have who present with these disorders.

Personality Disorders and a Medical Condition

> **Essential Points**
> - Many medical conditions can look like psychiatric disorders, in particular personality disorders.
> - Endocrine problems like hypothyroidism or hyperthyroidism may cause a patient to appear to have Paranoid or Borderline Personality Disorder.
> - Multiple sclerosis can cause personality changes that mimic Borderline, Narcissistic, Avoidant, or Dependent Personality Disorder.
> - AIDS patients can also seem to have personality disorders, i.e., borderline, histrionic, dependent, or narcissistic personality disorders.

Patients with medical conditions often have lowered self-esteem, feeling of hopelessness and helplessness, shame, anger, and increased dependency needs. They can regress and be in denial or isolate themselves. All of these symptoms may seem like personality disorders.

Many medical conditions change patients' moods and personalities. For instance, if a patient has Huntington's disease, she may be aggressive and paranoid. It may seem like she has Paranoid Personality Disorder, but she actually has increased dopamine production that causes the paranoia.

KEY POINT

The importance of proper medical and neurological evaluation becomes clear in patients who have sudden changes of mood or personality.

Endocrine problems like hyperthyroidism can make a patient look like he has a borderline personality if he suddenly is angry and fighting with everyone. In reality, his increased production of thyroid hormones makes him agitated. In hypothyroidism, the patient is slowed down, cranky, and can seem like a paranoid personality.

Multiple sclerosis, which causes demyelination of the spinal cord, has been associated with depression, mania, and personality changes. The reasons are not exactly known, but individuals with multiple sclerosis have been falsely diagnosed with borderline, narcissistic, avoidant, or dependent personality disorders. Perhaps so many defenses are evoked in this condition that patients appear to be enmeshed in personality disorders.

AIDS patients have also struggled to be free of being labeled borderline, histrionic, narcissistic, and dependent, when the cause of their mood changes was the HIV playing havoc with their brain chemistry. Many other infectious and inflammatory diseases like SLE, TB, and mononucleosis can cause psychiatric symptoms, which lead to false diagnoses.

Other neurological disorders, like Alzheimer's dementia, migraines, narcolepsy, and Wilson's disease, can make the doctors to believe patients have personality disorders when they do not.

Many medications or recreational drugs can also lead to false diagnosis of personality disorder.

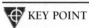 KEY POINT

Clinicians must always rule out these medical conditions before arriving at a final diagnosis.

Sometimes, psychiatrists are so positive that they are dealing with a personality disorder that they forget they have gone to medical school and they do not get a full chemical screen, thyroid function tests, a complete blood count, etc. Also they should demand that their patients get a thorough physical exam with an EKG.

CLINICAL VIGNETTE

Debbie, a physicist in her mid-thirties, hated to be identified with any women's issues. The only child of two chemistry professors she was raised to be an independent and scientific thinker. Between the ages of 8 and 13, she was a tomboy who enjoyed playing baseball and gazing at stars through a telescope in her backyard. At 14, menses began. Debbie tried to minimize the depressed and anxious moods that troubled her just before menstruation.

The moods were at least tolerable throughout adolescence. But in her twenties, Debbie noticed significant physical and mental changes in herself before menses. Her breasts would swell and ache, she developed migraines and her abdomen would bloat to the point where she could not wear her normal clothing. Debbie's moods were so bad that she would actually scream at colleagues. Even she was surprised at her own behavior. She was especially disturbed by her inability to concentrate. Usually, Debbie was even-tempered and logical, but just before her periods, she was distracted, fatigued, and out of control. Her sleeping was poor and she craved chocolate and junk food. Once her period actually began, she returned to a normal state.

Debbie disparaged herself for these premenstrual symptoms. The last thing she wanted was to fit the cliché about women being impossible during their periods, so she tried to hide her problems. She avoided her fiancé and friends a few days before each period. As much as she tried to stay away from people; however, she would inevitably get into an altercation with someone. Debbie endured her symptoms for many years until her fiancé broke up with her weeks before the wedding.

During a visit to her gynecologist, Debbie tearfully explained everything to the doctor who recommended that Debbie take Celexa 20 mg and visit a psychiatrist. Debbie agreed knowing she could not tolerate her life any longer.

To Debbie's surprise, her next period came and went almost unnoticed. Instead of feeling sad, hopeless, anxious, and angry, she felt fine from day 20 to 28 of her cycle, which was usually the worst time. She slept and ate normally and concentrated well. Her breasts and belly did not swell. Although she did get a migraine on day 26 of her cycle, her symptoms were remedied with the help of two aspirins.

In psychotherapy, Debbie came to understand that she had been denying her female issues. She operated under the belief that she was exactly the same as men she knew and that she did not have to adapt to her premenstrual dysphoric disorder (PDD). Debbie thought adapting would be akin to admitting that women were inferior.

Experiencing relief of PDD through medication allowed her to realize just how distressed she had been and to directly confront her unconscious prejudice against her own sex.

DISCUSSION

A total of 3% to 5% of women experience symptoms that meet the criteria of PDD. Most commonly, the disorder begins during the teens to late twenties and remits with menopause. Usually, women in their thirties like Debbie seek treatment.

PDD occurs during the luteal phase of menstruation, i.e., the time between ovulation and the onset of menses. Several studies have found an irregularity in serotonin, which may be why SSRIs like Celexa have been found effective in the treatment of PDD. Debbie's symptoms of depressed and anxious moods, affective lability, irritability, decreased interest in work and friends, difficulty concentrating, lethargy, and insomnia are all classical symptoms of PDD. Also in Debbie's case, they were mistaken for Borderline Personality Disorder and the cause for a breakup in her possible marriage. Medication cleared up her problem within a month. If she had had borderline or any other personality disorder, we would not have seen such a quick recovery.

Dimensional Models

Essential Concepts

- Many researchers and clinicians consider a dimensional model more useful for diagnosing personality disorders.
- The four personality traits considered are as follows:
  - Neuroticism/Negative Affect/Emotional Dysregulation
  - Extraversion/Positive Affect
  - Dissocial/Antagonism
  - Constraint/Compulsivity/Conscientiousness
- There is a movement to make a transition from the current DSM-IV-TR to a dimensional classification system.
- Some personality disorder patients would score high on one dimension and low on another.
- With a dimensional perspective, a diagnosis of a personality disorder would be an elevation of one or more of the traits listed above, plus dysfunction.

He's so frightened that he can't open any door to experience.

—A nurse on a psychiatric ward

The old-fashioned categorizing of personality disorders does not help us with predicting clinical outcomes or in treatment planning. Researchers and clinicians are concerned that the diagnosis of a personality disorder has a negative connotation and patients are treated poorly by doctors, hospitals, and insurance companies. There is also the problem of diagnostic reliability, co-occurrence, and inconsistent and arbitrary boundaries.

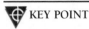 KEY POINT

Many say that there is inadequate scientific bases for the personality disorders. A good solution to the problem may be to look at various personality traits on a spectrum.

Does the patient have a negative or positive affect, is she extroverted or introverted, is he antagonistic or compliant, constrained or impulsive? There may be as many as 18 different models for a dimensional proposal. The four traits boiled down by Widiger et al. seem to work well in delineating the dimensions.

Many researchers are still arguing about how many factors are needed to represent differences in personality. Most people agree that the four dimensions of anxious-submissive, psychopathic, socially withdrawn, and compulsive are equivalent to neuroticism, disagreeableness, introversion/extraversion, psychoticism, and conscientiousness. Factor analysis has identified passive, dependent, sociopathic, anankastic, and schizoid features. Any classification system needs to score severity with any of these factors.

CLINICAL VIGNETTE

Cathy knew it was not a good sign that at age 50, she still lived with her mother. A robust, jovial train conductor, Cathy liked to boast to her many male coworkers about her great strength and physical health. She wished she could be as confident about her mental health.

After a short-lived marriage in her twenties, Cathy experienced a brief period of "freedom" that involved living alone, promiscuous sexuality, and development of a crack-smoking habit. Things progressively worsened into mania and her first hospitalization for which a diagnosis of bipolar disorder and Personality Disorder, Not Otherwise Specified (PDNOS) was made. Afterward, Cathy moved back in with her mother.

Although on the surface it appeared that the two women got along superbly, Cathy's younger brother knew the truth, having witnessed battles between them every time he visited, which now was not often. Cathy usually would awaken early, go diligently to work and return home late at night, except when her maternal relationship degenerated. At those times, she would isolate herself in her room and brood. Her social life was minimal.

After Cathy's second hospitalization for depression when she was 19, she was assigned a psychiatrist for weekly supportive psychotherapy. She began taking the mood stabilizer Depakote and antidepressant Celexa. Although she attended sessions as conscientiously as she went to work each day, it took a long time for her to reveal the physical and emotional abuse she had suffered at her mother's hands since childhood. She had never shared this information with anyone. Even worse, Cathy felt ashamed when her psychiatrist seemed surprised at her current living arrangements.

"How are you getting along with her now?" the doctor asked.

Cathy squirmed in her seat and wished she could give a different answer, but she had promised herself never to lie in therapy. She wanted to get better and believed that the truth would ultimately help her. "We fight all the time," she admitted.

"Wouldn't you be more comfortable living alone or with someone else?"

Cathy burst into tears. She had asked herself the same question for years, but there was something keeping her with the woman who disrespected her with snide remarks, slapped her in the face, and abused her in other small exasperating ways. "I'm working on moving out," Cathy promised—herself and the doctor.

As Cathy and her psychiatrist explored the issue, Cathy realized that although she felt great love for her mother, she basically disliked her. Her brother's way of dealing with the situation was avoidance because he blamed their father's early death from a heart attack on their mother's bickering and sadistic behavior.

Two months into treatment, Cathy was surprised to discover that she had developed a negative attitude toward her psychiatrist, although she had liked the doctor very much earlier in therapy. Even when the psychiatrist encouraged her to talk about these feelings, she could not. Instead, she missed several sessions and stopped taking her medication. She continued to attend work each day. One morning she found herself in an elated mood, but that quickly turned to hostility when her mother accused her of being "a lazy horse" and attempted to slap her. Suddenly, Cathy punched the 70-year-old woman in the face and ran out of the house. The police found her later, conducting her train, and forced her to enter the hospital for a third time.

DISCUSSION

In addition to having bipolar I disorder, Cathy had PDNOS. This diagnosis of PDNOS was carefully chosen by her psychiatrists to decrease the stigma which would have been greater if they would have called her a borderline personality or a passive-aggressive one or a dependent one or even a self-defeating personality. All of these personality disorders have a lot of negative qualities associated with them, whereas PDNOS is not that well known or despised as Borderline Personality Disorder is for example.

In a dimensional classification system, Cathy would be considered to be high on emotional dysregulation, low on extraversion (except when she was manic), high on antagonism, low on constraint, and high on conscientiousness. These scores would not stigmatize her. Also we can predict how she would react in the future and make better treatment plans to help her. Of course, her bipolar I disorder would have to be factored in to provide her with the best treatment.

32 ▼ Do They Ever Change?

Essential Points
- Do not expect therapies to change personality.
- Certain traits can be modified to change behavior with treatment.
- Identify which traits and behavior are maladaptive.
- Observe what emotions lead to what behaviors and try different techniques.
- Many times our patients do not have a happy ending to their problems.

> Given the characteristics of personality disorders (e.g., stable, resistant to change, difficult to treat) powerful treatments are required to achieve improvement.
> —*Handbook of Personality Disorders*, ed. Jeffrey Magnavita

We strive to have an adaptive ego that can respond to different stressors in a resilient way. Unfortunately, our personality disordered patients are either overcontrolled or undercontrolled. Both extremes are considered maladaptive.

Newer psychotherapies that have been tried for personality disorders are as follows: Cognitive Behavioral Therapy (CBT), Dialectical Behavior Therapy (DBT), Interpersonal Therapy (ITP), and Problem-Solving Therapy (PST). The more traditional therapies of psychoanalysis and psychodynamic psychotherapy have been used as well. Goal-focused group therapy is another one that is useful in personality disordered patients. Pharmacotherapy is necessary in many cases.

CBT is a relatively short-term, focused therapy that considers how the patient is thinking (cognitions), behaving, and communicating *today* rather than *yesterday* (in childhood). Studies show that CBT works well for depression, anxiety, OCD, phobias, and Axis I disorders. Therapists have attempted CBT with Axis II disorders and found that it takes longer, yesterday (childhood history) must be considered as well as transference issues. CBT starts with a basic assumption that moods and behavior are the products of thoughts. A stimulus causes a person to have an automatic thought (AT)—maladaptive ATs for personality disordered patients. These ATs cause physiological reactions, moods, and dysfunctional behaviors. The ATs originate in core beliefs (CBs). Most people with Axis I diagnoses have both positive and negative CBs, but most Axis II patients have mainly negative CBs. The deeply rooted negative CBs of our PD patients are ideas like, "I'm bad, I'm weak and helpless, I'm ugly and creepy." PD patients pay more attention to insults, which strengthens their CBs. Early childhood abuse forces PD patients into rigid patterns that are difficult to break. People with personality disorders get into treatment when they have an Axis I problem like anxiety or depression; however, their CBs need to be addressed so therapy takes longer and the therapist must be aware of therapist–patient interactions.

✪ KEY POINT

Many PD patients do not even have basic communication skills.

The clinician should not assume that the patients will understand the techniques that we teach them. Avoidant Personality Disorder patients will think "People will reject me," so they avoid them. They must examine their ATs about people and deal with their avoidance. The therapist helps the avoidant personality to imagine being accepted by people rather than rejected. It is extremely difficult for a PD patient to imagine other scenarios, rather than the familiar ones to which he is accustomed. Homework assignments will be ignored so therapy takes much longer. Borderline personality patients are especially difficult because of their early family environments that are dangerous and unstable. They see others as malignant and themselves as bad and powerless. When the CBT therapist works on the BPD patient, the first issue is to establish a relationship tolerant of the patient's ambivalence. Once this relationship is formed, the therapist must manage symptoms before any work can be carried out. Only then can ATs be addressed and CBs be identified. Treatment may be episodic as the patient tolerates and then rejects the therapist. The therapist must be flexible and adaptive—the opposite of the BPD patient.

DBT was originally developed by Linehan to treat patients with BPD. Research shows that it seems to be effective for patients with mood disorders or other personality disorders. DBT improves skills for emotional regulation by identifying and labeling emotions and increasing tolerance to distress as well as increasing positive emotions. A patient learns to be mindful, interpersonally effective, and to regulate emotions by recognizing them. Self-injurious and suicidal behaviors are first considered and then any behaviors that interfere with therapy. DBT skills are like assertiveness training. Patients learn to ask for what they need—they have a "dialogue" with the therapist or with a group. Especially useful are the tolerance behaviors that are taught. To survive, patients try to distract, self-soothe, improve the moment, or review through pros and cons.

ITP is a time-limited psychotherapy that developed in the 1970s for patients with unipolar depression. ITP has been used now for bipolar disorder, anxiety disorders, and even personality disorders. Psychodynamic theory is the parent of ITP, but ITP focuses on improving interpersonal skills. It is like CBT because it is time-limited and structured, but its concern is for the emotions not the cognitions. Also there is an emphasis on a supportive social network. For instance, a Narcissistic Personality Disorder patient may be asked to look at her current relationships to see how she views others. If she can gain awareness that others see her as selfish and ungiving, she can begin to accomplish some of the goals of ITP.

PST is a cognitive-behavioral clinical intervention in which patients adopt problem-solving attitude and skills. The idea is to enhance the quality of life and reduce psychopathology. It started in 1971 with D'Zurilla and Goldfried and then was refined by Nezu and Perri over the years. PST is based on research linking the psychosocial construct of social problem solving to psychopathology. People need to solve the problems of living by considering problem orientation and problem-solving style. If one considers problems a challenge it is better than considering them a threat and unsolvable.

Psychodynamic psychotherapy encourages the exploration of both conscious and unconscious emotional issues. It is one of the most common forms of therapy these days. It is not time-limited or structured. This type of therapy originated from classical psychoanalysis. Personality disordered patients benefit from the flexibility and adaptability of this form of therapy. Most patients are trapped in repetitive, maladapted patterns of reacting to others. Non–personality disordered patients can make more significant changes with this therapy, but even personality disordered patients can make some progress with psychodynamic psychotherapy.

Classical psychoanalysis grew out of hypnosis, in which the goals are remembering, abreaction, and the resolution of unresolved traumatic events. Many of our personality disordered patients' problems originated in the past, so one would think that psychoanalysis would be the treatment of choice. Many psychiatrists and other therapists have been attempting to use the tools of psychoanalysis on Axis II patients for over 100 years to no avail. The fundamental rule for the patient is to tell all—no holds barred—and the therapist is to listen with active free-floating attention but little interaction. A couch lends itself to this passivity. Psychoanalytical technique stresses that action based on impulse is to be avoided. Tell that to an impulsive histrionic or borderline patient. Free association, another basic tenet of psychoanalysis, will lose many a personality disordered patient. Transference is bound to be intense and unresolvable in many Axis II patients. Kohut and Kernberg are famous for analyzing "unanalysable" patients who were narcissistic or borderline.

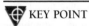 KEY POINT

Remember that the goal of psychoanalysis has always been to reorganize character structure by changing unhealthy defenses and inducing understanding in patients.

Nowadays, we do not expect any therapy to change personality. The newer therapies try to modify traits, like impulsivity or extraversion, and change behaviors.

The only patient I ever knew who decreased her borderline personality disorder traits went to a psychoanalyst for 4 years.

CLINICAL VIGNETTE

Adrian was 44 when she decided to use her hard-earned money, she worked as a secretary, to do psychoanalysis. I was skeptical, thinking that she would be better off joining a group or getting supportive therapy. She consulted with me for medication for her depression. I gave her Zoloft 100 mg per day, which treated her insomnia, blue moods, increased appetite, and suicidal thoughts. I saw her one time per month for years. Her depression went into remission but she continued in psychoanalysis two to three times per week, using the couch. At the beginning of treatment with me she was often nasty and hostile suspecting me of disliking her, which I did not. One week she would view me as all bad and her therapist as all good and then the next month I would be the "good one" and her therapist bad (uncaring and scheming). She often felt abandoned and had intense, unstable relationships with boyfriends and girlfriends. She was a binge eater and bulimic. Her anger was the worst to experience. She would be enraged if I did not return her nonemergency call within the hour and she had frequent displays of temper in my office. Over the 4 years that I knew her she "mellowed out." I attributed this change to her work in psychoanalysis. Her anger decreased considerably. She no longer felt abandoned. She did not fight with me or friends. People were not all good or bad. Her moods were stabilized I thought she had undergone an amazing transformation. I have never seen another patient so changed by therapy.

Pharmacotherapy is essential for PD patients suffering from major depression, bipolar disorder, psychotic disorders, and anxiety disorders. For major depression, we have SSRIs, e.g., Zoloft, Prozac, Celexa, Lexapro, Luvox, or TCAs like impramine. Effexor and Wellbutrin and Cymbalta are antidepressants that work on norepinephrine and dopamine systems. New antidepressants are always being developed. For bipolar patients, we often need mood stabilizers, i.e., Tegretol, Depakote, Topamax, etc., often combined with antidepressants. Antipsychotics include the older ones like Stelazine and Haldol as well as new ones, i.e., Abilify, Risperidal, Seroquel, etc. Antianxiety medications, like benzodiazepines, Klonopin, Xanax, and Valium, are useful. Many times, our PD patients have sleeping medications like Ambien or Rozerem for insomnia. We psychiatrists are the best doctors for determining medication needs.

Appendix

TABLE I. Characteristics of Personality Disorders

Personality Disorder	Socially Phobic	Psychotic	Feels In-adequate	Depressed	Anxious
Schizotypal	Yes	Maybe	No	Maybe	Yes
Schizoid	Yes	No	No	Maybe	Yes
Avoidant	Yes	No	Yes	Maybe	Yes
Paranoid	No	Maybe	No	Maybe	Maybe
Borderline	No	Maybe	Maybe	Maybe	Maybe
Narcissistic	No	No	No	Maybe	Maybe
Antisocial	No	No	No	Maybe	No
Histrionic	No	No	No	Maybe	Maybe
Dependent	Maybe	No	Yes	Maybe	Yes
OCD	No	No	Yes	Maybe	Maybe
NOS	Maybe	No	Maybe	Maybe	Maybe
Passive-Aggressive	Maybe	No	Yes	Maybe	Maybe
Self-defeating	Maybe	No	Yes	Maybe	Maybe

©2008 Carol W. Berman, M.D.

TABLE II. Diagnostic Criteria for 301.0 Paranoid Personality Disorder

A. A pervasive distrust and suspiciousness of others such that their motives are interpreted as malevolent, beginning by early adulthood and present in a variety of contexts, as indicated by four (or more) of the following:

    (1) suspects, without sufficient basis, that others are exploiting, harming, or deceiving him or her

    (2) is preoccupied with unjustified doubts about the loyalty or trustworthiness of friends or associates

    (3) is reluctant to confide in others because of unwarranted fear that the information will be used maliciously against him or her

    (4) reads hidden demeaning or threatening meanings into benign remarks or events

    (5) persistently bears grudges, i.e., is unforgiving of insults, injuries, or slights

    (6) perceives attacks on his or her character or reputation that are not apparent to others and is quick to react angrily or to counterattack

    (7) has recurrent suspicions without justification, regarding fidelity of spouse or sexual partner

B. Does not occur exclusively during the course of Schizophrenia, a Mood Disorder with Psychotic Features, or another Psychotic Disorder and is not due to the direct physiological effects of a general medical condition.

Note: If criteria are met before the onset of Schizophrenia, add "Premorbid," e.g., "Paranoid Personality Disorder (Premorbid)."

Reprinted with permission from the *Diagnostic and Statistical Manual of Mental Disorders*, Text Revision, 4th ed. (Copyright 2000). American Psychiatric Association.

TABLE III. Diagnostic Criteria for 301.20 Schizoid
Personality Disorder

A. A pervasive pattern of detachment from social relationships and
a restricted range of expression of emotions in interpersonal
settings, beginning by early adulthood and present in a variety
of contexts, as indicated by four (or more) of the following:
  (1) neither desires nor enjoys close relationships, including
  being part of a family
  (2) almost always chooses solitary activities
  (3) has little, if any, interest in having sexual experiences with
  another person
  (4) takes pleasure in few, if any, activities
  (5) lacks close friends or confidants other than first-degree
  relatives
  (6) appears indifferent to the praise or criticism of others
  (7) shows emotional coldness, detachment, or flattened
  affectivity
B. Does not occur exclusively during the course of Schizophrenia,
a Mood Disorder with Psychotic Features, another Psychotic
Disorder, or a Pervasive Developmental Disorder and is not due
to the direct physiological effects of a general medical
condition.

Note: If criteria are met before the onset of Schizophrenia, add "Premorbid," e.g.,
  "Schizoid Personality Disorder (Premorbid)."
Reprinted with permission from the *Diagnostic and Statistical Manual of Mental Disorders*,
  Text Revision, 4th ed. (Copyright 2000). American Psychiatric Association.

TABLE IV. Diagnostic Criteria for 301.22 Schizotypal Personality Disorder

A. A pervasive pattern of social and interpersonal deficits marked by acute discomfort with, and reduced capacity for, close relationships as well as by cognitive or perceptual distortions and eccentricities of behavior, beginning by early adulthood and present in a variety of contexts, as indicated by five (or more) of the following:
   (1) ideas of reference (excluding delusions of reference)
   (2) odd beliefs or magical thinking that influences behavior and is inconsistent with subcultural norms (e.g., superstitiousness, belief in clairvoyance, telepathy or "sixth sense"; in children and adolescents, bizarre fantasies, or preoccupations).
   (3) unusual perceptual experiences, including bodily illusions
   (4) odd thinking and speech (e.g., vague, circumstantial, metaphorical, overelaborate, or stereotyped)
   (5) suspiciousness or paranoid ideation
   (6) inappropriate or constricted affect
   (7) behavior or appearance that is odd, eccentric, or peculiar
   (8) lack of close friends or confidants other than first-degree relatives
   (9) excessive social anxiety that does not diminish with familiarity and tends to be associated with paranoid fears rather than negative judgments about self
B. Does not occur exclusively during the course of Schizophrenia, a Mood Disorder with Psychotic Features, another Psychotic Disorder, or a Pervasive Developmental Disorder.

Note: If criteria are met before the onset of Schizophrenia, add "Premorbid," e.g., "Schizotypal Personality Disorder (Premorbid)."

Reprinted with permission from the *Diagnostic and Statistical Manual of Mental Disorders*, Text Revision, 4th ed. (Copyright 2000). American Psychiatric Association.

TABLE V. Diagnostic Criteria for 301.7 Antisocial Personality Disorder

A. There is a pervasive pattern of disregard for and violation of the rights of others occurring since the age of 15, as indicated by three (or more) of the following:
  (1) failure to conform to social norms with respect to lawful behaviors as indicated by repeatedly performing acts that are grounds for arrest
  (2) deceitfulness, as indicated by repeated lying, use of aliases, or conning others for personal profit or pleasure
  (3) impulsivity or failure to plan ahead
  (4) irritability and aggressiveness, as indicated by repeated physical fights or assaults
  (5) reckless disregard for safety of self or others
  (6) consistent irresponsibility, as indicated by repeated failure to sustain consistent work behavior or honor financial obligations
  (7) lack of remorse, as indicated by being indifferent to or rationalizing having hurt, mistreated, or stolen from another
B. The individual is at least 18 years old.
C. There is evidence of Conduct Disorder with onset before the age of 15
D. The occurrence of antisocial behavior is not exclusively during the course of Schizophrenia or a Manic Episode.

Reprinted with permission from the *Diagnostic and Statistical Manual of Mental Disorders, Text Revision*, 4th ed. (Copyright 2000). American Psychiatric Association.

TABLE VI. Diagnostic Criteria for 301.83 Borderline Personality Disorder

A pervasive pattern of instability of interpersonal relationships, self-image, and affects and marked impulsivity, beginning by early adulthood and present in a variety of contexts, as indicated by five (or more) of the following:

(1) frantic efforts to avoid real or imagined abandonment. *Note*: Do not include suicidal or self-mutilating behavior covered in Criterion 5.

(2) a pattern of unstable and intense interpersonal relationships characterized by alternating between extremes of idealization and devaluation

(3) identity disturbance: markedly and persistently unstable self-image or sense of self

(4) impulsivity in at least two areas that are potentially self-damaging (e.g., spending, sex, substance abuse, reckless driving, binge eating). *Note*: Do not include suicidal or self-mutilating behavior covered in Criterion 5.

(5) recurrent suicidal behavior, gestures, or threats, or self-mutilating behavior

(6) affective instability due to a marked reactivity of mood (e.g., intense episodic dysphoria, irritability, or anxiety usually lasting a few hours and only rarely more than a few days)

(7) chronic feelings of emptiness

(8) inappropriate, intense anger, or difficulty controlling anger (e.g., frequent displays of temper, constant anger, recurrent physical fights)

(9) transient, stress-related paranoid ideation or severe dissociative symptoms

Reprinted with permission from the *Diagnostic and Statistical Manual of Mental Disorders, Text Revision,* 4th ed. (Copyright 2000). American Psychiatric Association.

TABLE VII. Diagnostic Criteria for 301.50 Histrionic Personality Disorder

A pervasive pattern of excessive emotionality and attention seeking, beginning by adulthood and present in a variety of contexts, as indicated by five (or more) of the following:

(1) is uncomfortable in situations in which he or she is not the center of attention

(2) interaction with others is often characterized by inappropriate sexually seductive, provocative behavior

(3) displays rapidly shifting and shallow expression of emotions

(4) consistently uses physical appearance to draw attention to self

(5) has style of speech that is excessively impressionistic and lacking in detail

(6) shows self-dramatization, theatricality, and exaggerated expression of emotion

(7) is suggestible, i.e., easily influenced by others or circumstances

(8) considers relationships to be more intimate than they actually are

Reprinted with permission from the *Diagnostic and Statistical Manual of Mental Disorders, Text Revision*, 4th ed. (Copyright 2000). American Psychiatric Association.

TABLE VIII. Diagnostic Criteria for 301.81 Narcissistic Personality Disorder

A pervasive pattern of grandiosity (in fantasy or behavior), need for admiration, and lack of empathy, beginning by early adulthood and present in a variety of contexts, as indicated by five (or more) of the following:

(1) has a grandiose sense of self-importance (e.g., exaggerates achievements and talents, expects to be recognized as superior without commensurate achievements)

(2) is preoccupied with fantasies of unlimited success, power, brilliance, beauty, or ideal love

(3) believes that he or she is "special" and unique and can only be understood by, or should associate with, other special or high-status people (or institutions)

(4) requires excessive admiration

(5) has a sense of entitlement, i.e., unreasonable expectations of especially favorable treatment or automatic compliance with his or her expectations

(6) is interpersonally exploitative, i.e., takes advantage of others to achieve his or her own ends

(7) lacks empathy: is unwilling to recognize or identify with feelings and needs of others

(8) is often envious of others or believes that others are envious of him or her

(9) shows arrogant, haughty behaviors, or attitudes

TABLE IX. Diagnostic Criteria for 301.82 Avoidant Personality Disorder

A pervasive pattern of social inhibition, feelings of inadequacy, and hypersensitivity to negative evaluations, beginning by early adulthood and present in a variety of contexts, as indicated by four (or more) of the following:

(1) avoids occupational activities that involve significant interpersonal contact, because of fears of criticism, disapproval, or rejection

(2) is unwilling to get involved with people unless certain of being liked

(3) shows restraint within intimate relationships because of the fear of being shamed or ridiculed

(4) is preoccupied with being criticized or rejected in social situations

(5) is inhibited in new interpersonal situations because of feelings of inadequacy

(6) views self as socially inept, personally unappealing, or inferior to others

(7) is unusually reluctant to take personal risks or to engage in any new activities because they may prove embarrassing

TABLE X. Diagnostic Criteria for 301.6 Dependent Personality Disorder

A pervasive and excessive need to be taken care of that leads to submissive and clinging behavior and fears of separation, beginning by early adulthood and present in a variety of contexts, as indicated by five (or more) of the following:

(1) has difficulty making everyday decisions without an excessive amount of advice and reassurance from others
(2) needs others to assume responsibility for most major areas of his or her life
(3) has difficulty expressing disagreement with others because of fear of loss of support or approval. *Note*: Do not include realistic fears of retribution.
(4) has difficulty initiating projects or doing things on his or her own (because of a lack of self-confidence in judgment or abilities rather than a lack of motivation or energy)
(5) goes to excessive lengths to obtain nurturance and support from others, to the point of volunteering to do things that are unpleasant
(6) feels uncomfortable or helpless when alone because of exaggerated fears of being unable to care for himself or herself
(7) urgently seeks another relationship as a source of care and support when a close relationship ends
(8) is unrealistically preoccupied with fears of being left to take care of himself or herself

TABLE XI. Diagnostic Criteria for 301.4 Obsessive-Compulsive Personality Disorder

A pervasive pattern of preoccupation with orderliness, perfectionism, and mental and interpersonal control, at the expense of flexibility, openness, and efficiency, beginning by early adulthood and present in a variety of contexts, as indicated by four (or more) of the following:

(1) is preoccupied with details, rules, lists, order, organization, or schedules to the extent that the major point of the activity is lost

(2) shows perfectionism that interferes with task completion (e.g., is unable to complete a project because his or her own overly strict standards are not met)

(3) is excessively devoted to work and productivity to the exclusion of leisure activities and friendships (not accounted for by obvious economic necessity)

(4) is overconscientious, scrupulous, and inflexible about matters of morality, ethics, or values (not accounted for by cultural or religious identifications)

(5) is unable to discard worn-out or worthless objects even when they have no sentimental value

(6) is reluctant to delegate tasks or to work with others unless they submit to exactly his or her way of doing things

(7) adopts a miserly spending style toward both self and others; money is viewed as something to be hoarded for future catastrophes

(8) shows rigidity and stubbornness

Reprinted with permission from the *Diagnostic and Statistical Manual of Mental Disorders, Text Revision*, 4th ed. (Copyright 2000). American Psychiatric Association.

Bibliography

Akiskal HS, Akiskal K. Cyclothymic, hyperthymic and depressive temperaments as subaffective variants of mood disorders. In: Annual Review of Psychiatry, vol II. Washington, DC: American Psychiatric Press, 1992.

American Psychiatric Association. Diagnostic and Statistical Manual of Mental Disorders. 4th Ed. Arlington, VA: APA, 2000.

Beck JS. Cognitive Therapy: Basics and Beyond. New York, London: Guilford Press, 1995.

Block JH, Block J. The role of ego-control and ego-resiliency in the organization of behavior. In: Collins WA, ed. Minnesota Symposium on Child Psychology, vol 13. Hillsdale, NJ: Lawrence Erlbaum, 1980:39–101.

Freud S. On narcissism. In: The Standard Edition of the Complete Psychological Works of Sigmund Freud, vol 14. London: Hogarth, 1914.

Gabbard GO. Cluster B personality disorders. In: Psychodynamic Psychiatry in Clinical Practice. 3rd ed. Washington, DC: American Psychiatric Press, 2000.

Goodwin DW, Guze SB. Psychiatric Diagnosis. New York: Oxford University Press, 1996.

Herman JL, Perry JC, van der Kolk BA. Childhood Trauma in Borderline Personality Disorder. Am J Psychiatry 1989;146: 490–495.

Kahn E. Psychopathic Personalities. New Haven: Yale University Press, 1931.

Kaplan H, Sadock B, Grebb J. Synopsis of Psychiatry. 7th Ed. Baltimore: Williams & Wilkins, 1994.

Kernberg OF. Borderline Conditions and Pathological Narcissism. New York: Aronson, 1975.

Kohut H. The Analysis of the Self. New York: International Universities Press, 1971.

Linehan MM, Dimeff L. Dialectical behavior therapy in a nutshell. The California Psychologist 2001;34(3):10–13.

Maj M, Akiskal H, et al: Personality Disorders. New Jersey: Wiley, 2005.

Nezu AM, Wilkins VM, Nezu CM. Social problem solving, stress and negative affective conditions. In: Chang EC, D'Zurilla TJ, Sanna LJ, eds. Social Problem Solving. Washington, DC: American Psychological Association, 2004.

Paris J. Personality Disorders over Time. Arlington, VA: APA, 2003.

Rothstein A. The Narcissistic Pursuit for Perfection. New York: International Universities Press, 1980.

Spitzer RL, Endicott J, Gibbon M. Crossing the border into border-line personality and borderline schizophrenia: the development of criteria. Arch Gen Psychiatry 1979;36:17–24.

Weissman MM, Markowitz JC. An overview of interpersonal psychotherapy. In: Markowitz J, ed. Interpersonal Psychotherapy. Washington, DC: American Psychiatric Press, 1998.

Widiger T, Simonsen E, Sirovatka, Regier D. Dimensional Models of Personality Disorders. Arlington, VA: American Psychiatric Association, 2006.

Index

A

Abilify, 53, 172
Abraham, Karl, 42
Adderall, 98
ADHD. *See* Attention-Deficit/Hyperactivity Disorder
Adolescence
Anorexia Nervosa and, 105
and appearance, 32
chronic depression and, 121
and conduct disorder, 96
and isolation, 37
moods and, 157
reminiscence of, 73
schizoid personality disorder and, 13
schizophrenia and, 86
and transition to adulthood, 48
Aggression, 102, 119
antisocial personality disorder and, 17, 66, 100, 120, 132, 147
bipolar disorder and, 71
conduct disorder and, 96
Huntington's disease and, 155
paranoid personality disorder and, 114
physical, 132
schizotypal personality disorder and, 114
See also Passive-aggressive personality disorder
Agnosia, 99
Agoraphobia, 78, 81
AIDS, 156
Alcoholism, 74, 115, 127, 136, 141, 142
Alzheimer's disease/dementia (AD), 67, 100, 101, 102

Ambien, 172
Amnesia, 103
Anger, 7, 19, 21, 22, 23, 55, 57, 67, 102, 107, 114, 127, 163, 172
Anhedonia, 66
Anorexia Nervosa, 105–107, 108
Antidepressants, 10, 27, 29, 33, 48, 69, 58, 75, 79, 92, 108, 115, 116, 172
See also individual entries
Antipsychotics, 9, 172
atypical, 87
Antisocial personality disorder (APD), 4, 17–20, 66, 119, 147–148
in ADHD patients, 96
Alzheimer's dementia and, 100
with Bulimia Nervosa, 107
clinical vignette, 18–19
discussion, 19–20
gender and, 131–132
low socioeconomic status and, 138
OCD and, 90
substance abuse and, 141–142
Anxiety, 19, 21, 24, 34, 149
and compulsions, 89
disorders, 77
medications for, 172
and schizotypals, 66
solving, 126
and temperament, 125
and thoughts, 43–44
Aphasia, 99
Apraxia, 99
Attention-Deficit/Hyperactivity Disorder (ADHD), 95–98
clinical vignette, 97–98

Auditory hallucination, 85, 86,
    135, 136
Authority, 45
    opposition to, 56, 57
Automatic thoughts, 168, 169
Avoidance. *See* Avoidant
        personality disorder
Avoidant personality disorder, 4,
        35–38, 61, 67, 78, 81, 126
    Alzheimer's dementia and, 101
    with Anorexia Nervosa, 106
    clinical vignette, 36–37
    cognitive behavioral therapy
        for, 168–169
    discussion, 37–38
    medical conditions, 127
    OCD and, 90
    substance abuse and, 142
Axis I (clinical disorder)
        diagnosis, 9, 10, 65, 66
    see also individual entries
Axis II (personality disorder),
        52, 72
    see also individual entries

B
β-blockers, 38
Behavior change, 167–172
    clinical vignette, 171–172
Benzodiazepines, 24, 38, 172
Bipolar disorder, 9, 71–75, 172
    bipolar I, 72, 73
    bipolar II, 72
    clinical vignette, 73
    discussion, 74–75
Borderline personality disorder
        (BPD), 4, 21–24, 67, 71,
        72, 78, 120, 148
    in ADHD patients, 96
    Alzheimer's dementia and,
        100
        clinical vignette, 101–102
        discussion, 102–103
    with Anorexia Nervosa, 106

[Borderline personality disorder]
    with Bulimia Nervosa, 107
    clinical vignette, 22–23
    countertransference feelings,
        123
    culture and, 139
    dialectical behavior therapy
        for, 169
    gender and, 132–133
    OCD and, 90
        clinical vignette, 91–92
        discussion, 92
    transference feelings, 122–123
BPD. *See* Borderline personality
        disorder
Bulimia Nervosa, 107

C
Caregivers, 39
CBT. *See* Cognitive Behavioral
        Therapy
Celexa, 48, 158, 159, 163, 172
Childhood, 32, 33, 42, 48, 53,
        55, 151
    abuse, 168
    antisocial, 132
    and avoidant personality
        disorder, 37
    and borderline personality
        disorder, 120
    and conduct disorder, 17, 96,
        119
    observation of, 125
    and SPD, 13, 15
    trauma and neglect in, 133
Chronic depression, 27, 121
Cluster A personality disorders,
        113–117
Cluster B personality disorders,
        119–123, 125–129
Cocaine, 127, 141, 142, 143,
        144, 145
Cognitive Behavioral Therapy
        (CBT), 34, 69, 168–169

Conduct disorder, 17, 96, 119
Constraint/compulsivity/conscie
        ntiousness, 164
Countertransference, 22
    borderline/narcissistic
        personality disorders
        and, 123
Culture, 36, 91, 133, 137–139
Cyclothymia, 74
Cymbalta, 172

D

DBT. *See* Dialectical Behavior
        Therapy
Deceit, 17, 119
Delusion, 72, 84, 86, 103, 113
Dementia, 99–103
    age of onset of, 100
    Alzheimer's disease/dementia
        (AD), 67, 100, 101, 102
    clinical vignette, 101–102
    discussion, 102–103
Depakote, 74, 163, 172
Dependent personality disorder
        (DPD), 4, 39–42, 67,
        126, 148
    Alzheimer's dementia and,
        101
    clinical vignette, 40, 127–129
    discussion, 41–42, 129
    gender and, 133–134
    medical conditions, 127
    OCD and, 90
    substance abuse and, 142
    with Anorexia Nervosa, 106
Depression, 10, 33, 34, 73, 74,
        75, 121, 127
    chronic, 27, 121
    and suicide, 116
    unipolar, 72, 75
    see also antidepressants; major
        depression
Dialectical Behavior Therapy
        (DBT), 169

Dimensional models, 15,
        161–165
Dissocial/antagonism, 164
Distress, 6, 44, 149, 150, 158,
        169
Distrust, 4, 8, 100
Down's syndrome, 103
DPD. *See* Dependent personality
        disorder
DSM-III-R, 61
DSM-IV-TR, 9, 15, 19, 23, 26,
        61, 84, 152

E

Eating disorders, 105–109
    clinical vignette, 107–109
    discussion, 109
Effexor, 128, 172
Emotional freezing, 138
Executive functioning,
        disturbance in, 99
Extraversion, 138, 164

G

Gender, 131–136
Group therapy, 37
goal-focused therapy, 167

H

Haldol, 172
Hallucination, 9, 72, 84
    auditory, 86, 135, 136
    visual, 101
Histrionic personality disorder
        (HPD), 4, 25–30, 67, 78,
        120, 148
    in ADHD patients, 96
    Alzheimer's dementia and,
        101
    with Anorexia Nervosa, 106
    with Bulimia Nervosa, 107
    clinical vignette, 26–29
    culture and, 137–138
    diagnosis, 26

[Histrionic personality disorder]
  gender and, 133
    clinical vignette, 134–135
    discussion, 135–136
  OCD and, 90
Hospitalization, 143
Hostility, 7, 20, 53, 55, 66, 71,
    114, 138, 164, 172
HPD. *See* Histrionic personality
    disorder
Huntington's disease, 155
Hyperthyroidism, 156
Hypomania, 71, 72
Hypothyroidism, 156

I

Imopramine, 172
Impulsivity, 17, 22, 23, 25, 46,
    66, 90, 96, 106, 120,
    142, 147, 171
  and Borderline personality
    disorder, 132–133
Interpersonal Therapy (ITP),
    169–170
Irritability, 21, 66, 72, 80, 144,
    148
ITP. *See* Interpersonal Therapy

K

Klonopin, 172

L

Lamictal, 74
Lewy Body Dementia, 101
Lexapro, 52, 53, 68, 92, 121,
    172
Lithium, 73, 74
Luvox, 172

M

Major depression, 10, 33, 65–69,
    72, 122, 172
  antidepressants, 58
  clinical vignette, 67–68

[Major depression]
  discussion, 68–69
  symptoms of, 116
Major Depressive Disorder, 90
Marijuana, 127, 141, 142
Masochism
  moral, 59, 61
  sexual, 59, 61
Mixed personalities, 47
Moods, 10, 22, 48, 72, 115, 157,
    168
  disorders, 116
  stabilizers, 74, 163, 172
Moral masochism, 59
Multiple sclerosis, 156

N

Narcissistic personality disorder
    (NPD), 4, 31–34, 67, 73,
    120, 148
  Alzheimer's dementia and,
    101
  with Anorexia Nervosa, 106
  with Bulimia Nervosa, 107
  clinical vignette, 32–33,
    148–150
  countertransference feelings,
    123
  discussion, 33–34, 150–151
  and Greek mythology, 31–33
  interpersonal therapy for,
    170
  OCD and, 90
  substance abuse and, 142
    clinical vignette, 143–145
    discussion, 145
  transference feelings, 122–123
Nardil, 127
Neuroticism, 138
Neurontin, 74
Nicotine, 141
Nocebo, 30
NPD. *See* Narcissistic personality
    disorder

O

Obsessive-Compulsive Disorder
(OCD), 89–93
Alzheimer's dementia and,
101
clinical vignette, 91–92
discussion, 92–93
Obsessive-compulsive
personality disorder
(OCPD), 4, 43–46, 67,
86, 87, 89–90, 96,
125–126, 148
with Anorexia Nervosa,
106–107
clinical vignette, 107–109
discussion, 109
with Bulimia Nervosa, 107
clinical vignette, 44–45
culture and, 137
discussion, 45–46
medical conditions, 127
Occupational functioning, 13
OCD. *See* Obsessive-Compulsive
Disorder
OCPD. *See* Obsessive-
compulsive personality
disorder
Opiates, 142
Oppositional Defiant Disorder,
58

P

Panic disorder, 77–81, 122
clinical vignette, 79–81
discussion, 81
PAPD. *See* Passive-aggressive
personality disorder
Paranoid personality disorder
(PPD), 4, 7–11, 66, 72,
78, 114, 148
Alzheimer's dementia and,
100
with Anorexia Nervosa, 106
with Bulimia Nervosa, 107

[Paranoid personality disorder]
clinical vignette, 8–9
diagnosis, 9–10
in minority
groups/immigrants/refuge
es, 138
OCD and, 90
substance abuse and, 142
Passive-aggressive personality
disorder (PAPD), 4,
55–58
clinical vignette, 56–57
discussion, 57–58
Paxil, 109, 121
PDD. *See* Premenstrual
dysphoric disorder
PDNOS. *See* Personality
Disorder, Not Otherwise
Specified
Persecutory delusions, 72
Personality change, 103
Personality disorder not otherwise specified (PDNOS),
4, 47–49, 163, 164
clinical vignette, 48
discussion, 48–49
Personality disorders, 3–6
ADHD and, 95–98
classifications, 4–5
clinical vignette, 5–6
and dementia, 99–103
eating disorders and, 105–109
and medical condition,
155–159
clinical vignette, 157–158
discussion, 158–159
and obsessive-compulsive
disorder, 89–93
substance abuse and, 141–145
clinical vignette, 143–145
discussion, 145
see also individual disorders
Personality traits, 5, 58, 137
types, 138, 161, 162

Pharmacotherapy, 27, 149, 167, 172
Placebo, 30
Posttraumatic stress order (PTSD), 147
  clinical vignette, 148–150
  discussion, 150–151
PPD. *See* Paranoid personality disorder
Premenstrual dysphoric disorder (PDD), 158
  clinical vignette, 157–158
  discussion, 158
Problem-Solving Therapy (PST), 170
Prozac, 108, 172
Psychiatrist, 3, 8, 15, 17, 61, 73, 75, 86, 109, 121–122, 123, 157, 164, 172
Psychoanalysts, 8, 17, 44, 170–171
Psychodynamic psychotherapy, 169, 170
Psychosis, 14, 84, 86, 87
Psychostimulants, 20
Psychotherapy, 3, 10, 14, 19, 27, 37, 54, 60, 69, 127, 128, 149, 158
  types, 167
Psychotism, 9, 14, 86, 138
PTSD. *See* Posttraumatic stress order

R
Resentment, 56, 57, 114
Risperdal, 73, 74
Risperidal, 172
Rozerem, 172

S
SADs. *See* Seasonal affective disorders

Sadism, 59, 164
Schizoid personality disorder, 4, 13–16, 46, 66, 78, 114, 115–117, 148
  Alzheimer's dementia and, 100
  with Anorexia Nervosa, 106
  with Bulimia Nervosa, 107
  clinical vignette, 14–15, 115–116
  criteria, 175
culture and, 139
  discussion, 15–16, 116–117
  OCD and, 90
  substance abuse and, 142
Schizophrenia, 9
  clinical vignette, 85–86
  discussion, 86–87
four A's of, 83
  symptoms, 83
Schizotypal personality disorder (SPD), 4, 51–54, 66, 75, 113, 114
  Alzheimer's dementia and, 100
  with Anorexia Nervosa, 106
  with Bulimia Nervosa, 107
  clinical vignette, 52–53
  comparison with schizoid personality disorder, 51–52
  discussion, 53–54
  OCD and, 90
  substance abuse and, 142
  in voodoo/shamanism, 139
Seasonal affective disorders (SADs), 74
Self-defeating personality disorder (SdPD), 4, 59–61, 97, 98
  clinical vignette, 60–61
  discussion, 61

Self-esteem, 39, 40, 80, 138
Seroquel, 172
Serotonin, 159
Sertraline, 14, 27
Sexual masochism, 59
Social phobia, 52
Somatoform disorders, 150–151
  clinical vignette, 151–152
  discussion, 152–153
Splitting, 21, 23
SSRIs, 38, 92, 150, 159, 172
Stelazine, 172
Substance abuse, 141–145
  clinical vignette, 143–145
  discussion, 145
Suspiciousness, 8, 9, 100

T
TCAs, 172
Tegretol, 74, 172
Topamax, 172
Transference, 27, 30, 168, 171

[Transference]
  borderline/narcissistic
      personality disorders
      and, 122–123
  establishing, 109

U
Unipolar depression, 72, 75

V
Valium, 172
Vascular dementia, 101

Y
Wellbutrin, 172
Withdrawal, 66, 67, 86, 100,
      103, 114, 127

X
Xanax, 172

Z
Zoloft, 29, 80, 149, 150, 171,
      172
Zyprexa, 86